Keeping in Touch

with someone who has Alzheimer's

JANE CRISP

Ausmed Publications

Melbourne

Australasian Health Education Systems Pty Ltd
(ACN 005 611 626)
trading as
Ausmed Publications
277 Mount Alexander Road
Ascot Vale, Victoria 3032, Australia

First published August 2000

Further copies of this book and of all other Ausmed publications are available from the Distribution Manager, Ausmed Publications,
PO Box 4086, Melbourne University, Parkville, Victoria 3052, Australia.
Telephone +613/(03) 9375 7311.
Fax +613/(03) 9375 7299.
E-mail ausmed@ausmed.com.au
Home page www.ausmed.com.au

National Library of Australia Cataloguing-in-Publication data:

Crisp, Jane.
Keeping in touch with someone who has Alzheimer's.

Includes index.
ISBN 0 9577988 2 2.

1. Alzheimer's disease - Patients. 2. Alzheimer's disease.
Title.

618.976831

Edited by Robyn Whiteley and John Collins, The WC Company Pty Ltd
Cover, design, typesetting and printing by Hyde Park Press, 4 Deacon Avenue, Richmond, South Australia 5033, telephone (08) 8234 2044, fax (08) 8234 1887, e-mail hpp@olis.net.au

Text set in 11/14 Slimbach

Cover: The author with her mother, Bettie, and Bettie's friend Wally

FOREWORD

When Jane Crisp's mother entered the world of dementia, Jane saw this not as a tragedy, but as a challenge and a wonderful new opportunity for communication with her deeply loved mother. Out of that very positive approach has grown this book, one of the most remarkable books ever written about dementia.

For too long, and purely as a result of misinformation, we have been quite cruel to people with dementia. We believed that dementia meant that they had become mindless and it was impossible to establish real understanding with them. So we talked about them as if they could not hear what we were saying; we talked pleasantly to them or even asked questions, but then never listened for the answer. Worst of all, we stopped talking to them, saying to ourselves 'they are quite past it'. This total misunderstanding of dementia arose out of the false concept of dementia as a disease.

It is now clear that, although dementia has its basis in some kind of damage to the brain tissue, it is actually just a state of being in which people become confused, but carry with them their past culture and experience, their personal sense of who they are, an understanding of and response to their social environment, and a great deal of their life resources.

If we can totally reject the old misunderstandings, and treat affected people still as full people, with minds of their own, who are entitled to the total respect of others, then people with dementia can live full and satisfying lives. More importantly, they can still share their lives with us.

This book is Jane's story of a joyful journey with her ageing mother — a journey of love, continuing understanding and the excitement of discovering new ways of being close to each other. But the story is told so that we can all share in that journey and use the guideposts which Jane and her mother discovered to make similar journeys with our own loved ones.

In the book Jane moves to and fro between her personal journey, on one hand, and her sense of rigorous intellectual inquiry on the other. It is this merging of personal experience with a research perspective that makes her book so extraordinary. My own journey into the world of dementia has been research-based and although that has given me a sense of just how wrong our traditional concepts have been, it was crossing paths with Jane that enriched my understanding immensely, and brought me to recognise and fully accept the continuing social capacities of people with dementia.

I am delighted to invite you all to share in our journey from your perspective, whether it be as a family member or as a professional carer. Open your mind to really hear people with dementia, and I am certain you can find it just as rewarding and exciting as we have.

Elery Hamilton-Smith.

Elery Hamilton-Smith
Professor
Lincoln Gerontology Centre
LaTrobe University, Melbourne, Australia

CONTENTS

ACKNOWLEDGMENTS

First, I wish to thank the countless family and professional carers who have shared their experiences with me over the years and encouraged me to continue with the project which has led to this book. The names of many of you are unknown to me, because we met in passing on social occasions or at conferences. Others, however, whose encouragement and support have sustained me throughout, I am fortunately able to acknowledge individually here.

Thanks are due to Griffith University, Brisbane, for the grant that initially made possible a change in the direction of my research and for the periods of study leave that gave me the opportunity to develop my new project and, more recently, to write *Keeping in Touch*.

I owe a special debt of gratitude to the friends and colleagues that I have gained in the fields of psycho-gerontology, neurology and professional caregiving in France and Belgium. Dr Louis Ploton, of the University Lumiere-Lyon, invited me to a key colloquium of dementia specialists at Lyon and put me up in the Jardin d'Eleusis home of which he was then director. On that occasion I met Dr Natalie Rigaux, from the Faculty of Sociology, Notre-Dame-de-la-Paix, Namur, Belgium. Her ongoing friendship, hospitality, and readiness to read and discuss my work with me have been immensely helpful to me.

Many thanks are due also to Dr Thomas de Broucker, of the Neurology Section of Hospital Delafontaine, St Denis, France, and to Dr Gilles Fenelon of the Neurology Section of Hospital Tenon, Paris, and members of their teams, especially Marie-Josee Manifacier-Fournier, psychologist at Hospital Tenon, and Isabelle Vendeuvre, speech therapist, at Hospital Vaugirard, Paris, for the many stimulating roundtable discussions in which we have shared ideas.

Dr Mitra Khosravi, psychologist and educator/consultant for family carers, is another person whose friendship and readiness to share ideas have added greatly to my periods of study leave in Paris; she also provided some of the specific examples quoted in this book. Many thanks also to Yves Christen,

Director of the IPSEN Foundation (Fondation IPSEN) for therapeutic research, Paris, and editor of *Alzheimer Actualités*, for access to their archives and for his ongoing encouragement. I am also extremely grateful to Claude Cusset and to Arnaud Fraisse, immediate past and present directors of France Alzheimer, Paris, for access to their resources and for their kindly encouragement too.

Other French-speaking specialists to whom I owe especial thanks are Dr Frederic Aumjaud, psychiatrist, for his hospitality and for introducing me to the psycho-gerontological world of Angers; Loic Laine, then runner of 'memory workshops' in Angers and now enjoying his active retirement in Brittany; Annette Arnaud, head of nursing at Haut Mitry, Nantes; Nicole Gardiol, visiting physiotherapist at residential care centres in and around Geneva; Yves Ledanseurs, founder-director of Memoire et Vie, Sucy-en-Brie, for the invitation to participate in a workshop series for professional carers at which I met Annette Arnaud and Nicole Gardiol; and Marie Constant-Troussard, physiotherapist, for the privilege of attending one of her workshops for people with dementia at the Forum Vignalou, Hospital Charles Foix, Paris.

Thanks are also due to Clive Evers, in charge of Information and Training at the Alzheimer's Disease Society in London, and to Dr Charlotte Clarke, of the Faculty of Health, Social Work and Education, University of Northumbria at Newcastle, for encouraging me to go ahead with a book for family carers.

Amongst my Australian colleagues, special mention should be made of Professor Judith Parker of La Trobe School of Nursing, and of Associate Professor Elery Hamilton-Smith, Lincoln Gerontology Centre, for their kind support and encouragement over the years; and also of Dr Helen Chenery, Department of Speech and Hearing, University of Queensland, for sharing the response to the sketch of a beaver quoted in chapter 1.

In New Zealand I have to thank Anne Crawford and Robyn Thomas, professional carers, for sharing ideas with me. My love and deep gratitude too to Olwen and Neil Laurie, close friends of my mother to the end.

Very special thanks are due also to my family: to my father, for entering so thoroughly into the spirit of my project and for sharing his experiences, both positive and negative, through the long final years of my mother's life, and to Colin, my husband, for the encouragement and intelligent readership that have sustained me throughout.

Finally, my greatest debt of gratitude is to the person without whom this project would never have begun — Bettie, my mother. *Keeping in Touch* is dedicated to her memory.

A NOTE ON THE USE OF TERMS

Health professionals using this book will be aware that there is a problem concerning the term 'Alzheimer's disease'. Although this is the term used most widely to refer to the typical cluster of symptoms described in chapter 2, strictly speaking, Alzheimer's disease refers only to cases where there are physical changes in the brain tissue of the sort originally described by Alois Alzheimer. These changes are, in many cases, verifiable only by autopsy, and, interestingly, are not always accompanied by the actual symptoms of dementia. Moreover, these symptoms themselves could be produced by any one of a very wide range of physical and even psychological causes or by several of these acting together. Hence, a medical diagnosis made during the person's lifetime will usually be one of *probable* Alzheimer's disease. Another problem too is that the condition described by Alzheimer is not, so far as we know, a 'disease' in the medical sense.

For these reasons, Kitwood[i] and many other specialists on dementia and dementia care prefer to use the more general term 'dementia', since this clearly identifies the person's symptoms without specifying their cause. However, because Alzheimer's disease is still the term that most family carers recognise I decided to employ it here in a book which has been written primarily for them. What I have done, though, is to employ 'dementia' equally throughout. More importantly, I have deliberately chosen to avoid such expressions as 'dementia sufferer' and even 'Alzheimer's patient', because these emphasise the medical condition rather than the person. Instead, I refer to 'people with dementia' and 'people like my mother' so as to underline the central point that I am trying make — these really are still people with whom we can stay in touch.

INTRODUCTION

HOW THIS BOOK BEGAN —
KEEPING IN TOUCH WITH MY MOTHER

A lifelong friendship

I wrote this book because of my mother. She and I were always very close. Her only child, I was born in England at the beginning of the war and was her chief companion throughout my father's long absences on military service. Our closeness continued after the war, when the family migrated to New Zealand, and throughout my school and university years. Even when I married and was living and working overseas my mother was still a very special and much-loved friend. We kept in touch by means of letters and frequent visits. My husband and I and our son would often spend the summer holidays with my parents in New Zealand, and they in turn would come to us in Australia for several weeks at a time. Throughout, my mother continued to share my interests and support my various projects: she hunted enthusiastically in junk shops for novels by the nineteenth century woman authors on whom I was working and she loved to make clothes for me, as she had since I was a child. (I still have and wear some of these clothes. My mother would often use French original patterns to stunning effect.)

In June 1986 we celebrated my mother's eightieth birthday together. Our son arranged for eighty gas-filled balloons to be delivered to the house in honour of the occasion — much to my mother's delight, as she adored balloons and, as she said, had never until then had enough of them to satisfy her. By then, though, my mother was becoming increasingly forgetful of recent events. She still enjoyed many of her old pleasures, but there were more and more things that she needed help with or could no longer do — finishing a simple blouse took weeks rather than a day, and her favourite rockeries were starting to look overgrown and neglected. Eventually these symptoms were officially diagnosed as being due to the onset of Alzheimer's disease.

Coping with Alzheimer's disease

My father and I were extremely worried about what the future had in store.

Given the inevitable and serious effects of dementia of the Alzheimer's type, would we be able to provide the increasing care that my mother would need? Would she change beyond recognition from the person we had known and loved for so long? And would we be able to maintain anything like our previously close relationships with her?

However, we discovered, as many other family members and professional carers of people with Alzheimer's disease have done, that, **despite the changes caused by dementia, more of the person survives than we expect.** Hence we were able to maintain a real relationship with my mother, up to and beyond the stage when we reluctantly had to admit her into full-time professional care. (My father's age and lack of physical strength, together with my family and work commitments overseas, finally made this decision unavoidable.)

Like other carers, we discovered that **maintaining a relationship with someone who has Alzheimer's is often hard work,** and requires not only willingness to make the effort, regardless of discouragements, but also a fair degree of imagination and ingenuity in coming up with strategies to compensate for the other person's problems and to make our contact with them worthwhile.

My mother died in June 1996 at the age of ninety, five and a half years after her admission to full-time professional care. And yes, despite the progressive changes in what she could say, do and remember, my father and I were able to keep in touch with her right up to the end of her life.

Sharing strategies with other carers

My personal knowledge of my mother and the fact that we had always been close were obviously crucial factors in my being able to keep in touch with her during these final years. However, I realised that another important factor was ideas about communication and language, with which I was familiar from my years of study and teaching at university. This professional knowledge gave me additional help in understanding and relating to my mother, and even provided me with strategies for making sense of the increasingly confused and fragmented things that she was saying. Out of this combination of personal experience and professional knowledge arose the more general project of helping other carers to understand and communicate with people who have Alzheimer's disease. Since my mother had always been enthusiastically involved in my previous research projects, it is appropriate that this project too should be one that so intimately involved her and that would have been impossible — unthinkable even — without her. This book is dedicated to her.

FOR PEOPLE WHO WANT TO KEEP IN TOUCH

Wanting to keep in touch

This book is for people who find themselves in the same situation as my father and I did — someone close to you (your spouse, your parent, a dear friend) has been diagnosed as having Alzheimer's disease and you want to keep in touch with them as long as you possibly can. This desire to stay in touch may be because you love them, or feel a sense of duty or responsibility towards them; probably it will be a mixture of both. You'll be relying on these feelings of love and responsibility to carry you through the times ahead, whatever the circumstances.

The person with whom you want to keep in touch may be living with you. Later they may well be in full-time residential care, as my mother eventually was. The suggestions in this book apply to either situation. Some people who want to keep in touch may, like me, be living at a distance and have other responsibilities to fulfil. If so, the strategies in this book should still help you make best use of any time you can spend visiting a family member or friend who has dementia. There are also some suggestions about how you can maintain a sense of contact during the periods when you are absent.

Many professional carers should also find this book useful, given the increasing emphasis on the need to treat people with dementia as people and to meet their social and emotional needs as well as their physical ones.

Even if you don't want to, it may be worth trying

Not everyone will want to keep in touch with a family member who has Alzheimer's disease. If you have never been particularly close to the person in question, now will scarcely seem the moment to try. Indeed, any existing problems in your relationship will almost certainly be aggravated by the effects of their dementia on you both.

However, it is worth bearing in mind that a number of carers have actually developed a better rapport with their family member than they had with them before the onset of Alzheimer's. Some carers, for instance, find that apparent coldness and indifference crumble away, allowing an earlier, more affectionate self to emerge. This gives them an unexpected but welcome last chance to develop a more satisfactory relationship. The strategies suggested in this book should help you to establish some sort of relationship, if you do want to try. If not, there are other ways of fulfilling any obligation that you may have — such as providing financial and other practical forms of support for whoever may be taking on the burden of primary care.

WHAT 'KEEPING IN TOUCH' MEANS IN THIS BOOK

It means continuing to be in contact with the other person and to interact positively with them. It can mean simply being there for them as a friendly presence, as someone who cares. This is the essence of keeping in touch with anyone, whether they have dementia or not.

Keeping in touch is possible, despite the inevitable changes

Keeping in touch in this basic sense is possible with someone who has Alzheimer's disease, even though your interactions with them will gradually change.

You will find that they become less able to engage in exactly the same sort of conversation or activity that you once enjoyed together. My mother, for example, gradually forgot the Jane Austen novels that had previously been a constant point of reference between us. Sharing with them any new interests that you now have may become less possible. They may be unable to recall what you have told them about your recent life, and hence, generally speaking, may seem less concerned about your doings than they once were; they may well eventually forget your name or call you by the name of someone else in the family.

Despite such changes, the essentials of many previous interests that you had in common will survive. My mother and I still shared a love of gardens and animals, and a pleasure in words. Her liking for teddy bears survived too and was to prove an invaluable source of playful interactions between us. And even when my mother became unsure of my exact name, she still had a sense of my basic identity as a much-loved and *very important person* (these were her own words, during my last visit to her, in reply to a passer-by who asked who I was).

What counts most is being in touch — still giving attention to and responding to each other — however simple or minimal the content of our interactions becomes.

The physical side of keeping in touch

Keeping in touch is also a matter of physical contact, of being literally close to someone. This was one reason for choosing 'keeping in touch' to sum up what this book is about. An essential part of the pleasure of being with a friend or with someone whom we love is their warm, friendly presence — the familiar look of them, the sound of their voice. We can hold hands, exchange loving hugs, offer a supportive arm when walking together.

I always had a very warm physical relationship with my mother. Touching her, hugging her, helping her with personal grooming were things that I felt comfortable about doing; and these were to become invaluable as a way of maintaining contact with her. Even if your own relationship with your family member or friend was previously not a demonstrative one, you will find that touch becomes more and more important. You will be touching the other person when you are giving them the help and care that they will require; moreover, you will find that more and more they will need the basic reassurance that friendly human contact gives.

Given the increasing importance of physical contact with someone in my mother's condition, there is no substitute for being able to spend time with them in a routine, regular and informal way. I regretted the fact that I lived too far away to be able to help my parents on a daily basis. However, there are ways of keeping alive the other person's sense of you as someone who cares about them, especially if there is someone on the spot who is happy to co-operate in this. When I did visit, I made sure that I was there for at least a week so that I could be company for my mother as I had been on visits home in the past, rather than just someone dropping in to see her in passing.

Keeping in touch with someone you know

We usually want to keep in touch with someone because we know and like them — they are 'our sort of person'. Once they have Alzheimer's disease, though, our feeling of still knowing them may well be threatened. They forget things that formerly interested you both. Similarly, changes in their behaviour and in the way they use words make it more difficult to understand them or to see them still as the person they were. However, if we learn to look beyond the changes produced by their dementia we will realise that more of the essential person survives than we might expect. We can draw upon our personal knowledge of their past life and interests to help us recognise and reinforce these surviving elements.

But *as well as recognising their past self we also need to have some insight into the person that they are now.* After all, most people do change and develop over the years, so keeping in touch with someone usually includes catching up on their present self as well as reminiscing about the past. We can do this with someone who has Alzheimer's if we bother to spend time with them and listen to what they are saying.

Keeping in touch over the years

We expect keeping in touch with any friend to involve maintaining contact with them over a long period of time. We need to bear this in mind in the case of someone who has Alzheimer's disease, since they may well live for another seven to ten years after being diagnosed. But being with and caring for someone with dementia is often difficult and exhausting so we must take stock of what we will be able to sustain in the long term. *If we begin by setting an impossible standard for ourselves, refusing all help and trying to be there for them all day, every day, we will end up exhausting ourselves.* Any negative feelings we may have about the person and the burden of caring for them — feelings which even the most loving and devoted of carers are bound to experience from time to time — become stronger and more frequent. We come to resent the time, energy — and money — that caring for someone with Alzheimer's involves and wish that they would hurry up and die. And these feelings, and our guilt about having them, exhaust us even further.

My father cared for my mother as long as he was able to, first at home and then in sheltered accommodation attached to the hospital to which she was finally admitted for full-time care. Much as he hated to admit defeat (he has always been a doer and an achiever) he recognised that there were limits to what he could do for my mother if he wanted to last the distance for her. Because he was on the spot he could keep in touch by visiting her each morning, but he also had his own writing project to which he gave time each day and which, he said, 'helps keep me sane'. I had family and work commitments in Australia but I made extended visits to my parents, either alone or with my husband, whenever possible. While I was there I could afford to spend most of each day with my mother, and my father took this as an opportunity to have a break from regular visiting. We also persuaded him to come to stay with us occasionally for several weeks, although he would do this only at times when other close friends were able to make frequent visits to my mother in his place.

In an ideal world, and with unlimited money and energy, we could probably have done more for my mother than we did. But by learning to accept the limits of what we could manage to do, both of us were able to last the distance and to keep in touch with her, regardless of occasional setbacks and bad days, right up to the end.

Being realistic about what you can manage to do

What you can manage to do, then, will depend on you — your health, your family and other commitments, your financial circumstances, and the type of relationship that you already have with the person who now has dementia. The choices you make should be ones that suit you as an individual, that allow you to 'last the distance'. Be realistic about what you can sustain over an extended period — caregiver burnout is recognised as a serious problem in caring for people who have Alzheimer's and looking after the health and wellbeing of the carers themselves is a major priority for support organisations such as the Alzheimer's Association.

THE VALUE OF KEEPING IN TOUCH

Looking back

Keeping in touch takes time and effort but it is enormously valuable for all concerned. Now that my mother is dead I can look back and be grateful that I was able to do something for her, and that we stayed good friends and companions to the last. Instead of needing to blot out the last seven years or so to preserve the memory of the mother who meant so much to me, I have an additional store of memories from this final period. I recall the stories that she told me, the songs we sang together loudly in a private corner of the hospital garden, the fun we had with Growler, her teddy bear. Many of these memories I will be sharing with you in the course of this book, together with the memories and experiences of other carers who have found that it is possible to keep in touch.

Helping their sense of self to survive

The efforts that we make to keep in touch are also enormously valuable for the person with dementia. We all 'need a little help from our friends'; we depend on our contact with other people to maintain our sense of identity and self-worth, especially when these are under threat. This applies with even more force to people with Alzheimer's, who are not only burdened with the symptoms of dementia but risk being treated as if they are less than fully human because of this.

Alzheimer's disease has been described as causing 'a living death' and 'the loss of self'. However a number of recent studies have stressed that these terms are misleading. As Sabat and Harre[ii] have demonstrated, someone with Alzheimer's doesn't lose their personal self. This continues to be expressed through the use of the words 'I', 'me' and 'my' and of gestures that say the same thing — 'this chair, this cardigan, this plate of food is mine'.

What they do often lose, however, is their social self. Our social self or identity depends for its existence on being recognised by other people. What others say to us, how they behave towards us, confirms us in our role as their parent, child, teacher, student, colleague, etc. Their behaviour also expresses the value that we have for them in that role, telling us that we are, for instance, a much-loved parent, or merely a dogsbody. Someone with Alzheimer's needs us to treat them as a person of value, but sometimes we fail to co-operate. *If we ignore them, talk about them as if they weren't there, treat them as if they are a member of the living dead, we are showing them that they no longer have a valid social identity in our eyes.*

A positive role for carers

Even though Alzheimer's disease is, to date, largely incurable, we can do a great deal to help someone with it feel that they are still a person of value. *We cannot abolish their symptoms, but we can lessen the effects of these and help to make their life more worth living.* Our own work as carers becomes more rewarding too when it is not just a matter of keeping a body fed, clean and quiet but also a matter of recognising and supporting a fellow human being. In addition, the affection and respect that we show towards the person for whom we care has the advantage of giving them more status in the eyes of others and increasing their chances of being treated as someone of worth by them.

CHAPTER 1
BEING POSITIVE

WHAT THIS CHAPTER COVERS

The overall aim of this chapter is to help you to think in more positive terms about someone with Alzheimer's disease. This prepares the ground for the strategies for keeping in touch that are described in later chapters.

- *First I'll deal briefly with the highly negative picture of Alzheimer's disease which sometimes prevents people from interacting positively with someone who has the condition. To counteract this we need to keep sight of the person, rather than the disease.*

- *The rest of the chapter helps us to do this by emphasising the many things that someone who has dementia can still do, despite the effects of their condition.*

LOOKING BEYOND THE NEGATIVE PICTURE OF ALZHEIMER'S DISEASE

An added burden — the negative side of the picture

If you care for someone who has Alzheimer's one of the first problems that you have to cope with is the extremely negative picture usually given of this condition. So black are the terms in which it is described that it may be hard to believe that anything of the person you have known and loved will survive for long. Even in otherwise helpful books about the condition, dementia of the Alzheimer's type is described as a 'loss of self' and a 'living death'. Similarly, accounts in the media about well-known public figures with Alzheimer's disease — the former American president, Ronald Reagan; the glamorous film star, Rita Hayworth; the distinguished English novelist, Iris Murdoch; the Australian journalist, Claudia Wright — tend to draw a tragic contrast between the person they once were and what they have become.

Medical accounts of Alzheimer's disease also emphasise the negative. What is relevant from a clinical point of view is diagnosing the condition and charting its progress. Hence what gets listed and measured are the various problems and deficits that are symptoms of dementia.

These negative pictures are understandable, given the serious and progressive effects of dementia and the fact that (so far) the condition is incurable. However, they offer little help or comfort to someone who wants to keep in touch with a much-loved parent, spouse or friend. I well remember my own feelings of growing despair when I was first reading about Alzheimer's disease in hopes of learning something that would help me and my father cope with whatever was in store for us.

Because of this, one thing I will not be doing in this book is dwelling on the negative. Instead I will be stressing the positive — the capacities that survive in someone with Alzheimer's and the strategies that you can use to make the most of your time together.

Seeing the person instead of the disease

Fortunately, many carers, both professional and family, have succeeded in moving beyond the negative. Instead of losing sight of the 'person behind the disease', they continue to recognise and value all those human and endearing qualities which can and do survive even into the final stages of dementia.

- Despite the many symptoms of her condition, my mother remained someone whom I could relate to and love. She still had feelings and could express them; she was still trying to understand what was going on around her; she still had a sense of humour; she could make friends and interact with other people; and she still appreciated my company — even though she no longer knew what year it was or who the current prime minister was. Naturally, I wish that my mother had never had Alzheimer's disease, but we still had plenty of good times together for all that, in the years between her diagnosis and her death.

- Seeing the person rather than their disease is the best answer to the vexed question of whether someone with Alzheimer's disease is 'still the person that they once were'. Because the symptoms of dementia are so obvious, and increasingly serious in their effects, it is easy to regard the person as radically changed and even as being no longer a person. One doctor gave the following advice to my father: *'This is no longer the woman that you once knew and loved — forget about her and get on with your own life.'* The advice was well-meaning, and if my father had ceased to care for my mother, it might have been a help. As it was, however, it upset him deeply. Other carers have received similar advice and been similarly hurt by it.

• Many apparent changes are probably due to a loss of inhibition and hence a greater readiness to show feelings than before. What we are experiencing therefore may not be a different person but someone closer to the inner self that was previously hidden behind a veneer of social politeness and self-protection. Frena Gray-Davidson makes the helpful suggestion that what emerges from behind this veneer is 'the child in all of us'.[iii] Someone with Alzheimer's often speaks and behaves like a child, and as a result may be infantilised or treated dismissively by others. However, we will be much less likely to react in this way if we acknowledge that we carry a similar child-self inside us too — in our case it is just better hidden!

• Even though dementia of the Alzheimer's type has a characteristic set of symptoms, which are shared by people with this condition, each person is affected differently — they remain individuals, despite their common diagnosis.

> My mother's good friend Wally had only a few stock phrases and ended up scarcely able to speak at all, whereas my mother was someone for whom words had always been important, and she continued to respond to the stimulus of engaging in conversation with us. Our readiness to talk to her and to listen to what she had to say undoubtedly helped to keep this key aspect of her personality alive.

• The question of whether someone with Alzheimer's keeps their basic personality or not can also be explained in terms of the particular aspects of personality that we are giving priority to in forming our opinion on this matter. If we value someone for their sharp mind and their ability to organise and get things done, we will be likely to see their dementia as having caused a radical change in them. However, if what we value are the more emotional and imaginative aspects of their personality, we will probably still recognise these qualities in them and find it easier to relate to them as before.

John Bayley's recent account of his marriage to Iris Murdoch provides a striking example of this.[iv] Even though Alzheimer's disease had robbed his wife of the intellectual skills on which her distinguished career as a novelist had depended, she was still someone special; her goodness, her sense of humour and her 'old gentleness' continued to inspire his admiration and love.

It is easier to cope with Alzheimer's disease in someone for whom we care if we give full value to the person that they are now rather than fretting endlessly over what is no longer possible for them.

RECOGNISING WHAT SOMEONE WITH ALZHEIMER'S CAN STILL DO

Demonstrating the other side of the picture

As a French friend once remarked, when I asked politely about her chronically bad health, *'Think of it this way — you can think of your bottle of wine as half empty or you can think of it as half full.'* The following example demonstrates that there are indeed two ways of thinking about someone with Alzheimer's disease — not in terms of what they have lost, but in terms of what they can still do.

A common symptom of dementia is having problems giving objects their correct name. This symptom is exploited in a standard test (known as the Boston Naming Test) which is used to diagnose the condition and its severity. The person being tested is shown a series of simple line drawings and asked to give the correct one-word name for the items shown. A man with Alzheimer's who was being tested by Helen Chenery, a linguist at the University of Queensland, gave the following response to a sketch of a beaver:

'Fish — no it's not a fish. I've seen it on TV. Rat — no it's not a rat.'

Strictly speaking this response was wrong. However, as Helen and I agreed, what makes it interesting is everything that was actually right about it! Indeed, it has been seriously suggested that diagnostic tests like this one should be marked on the basis of how appropriate the replies are, rather than on a simple right/wrong basis, if we want to evaluate people with dementia more fairly.

- His response shows that the person was interacting with his questioner — and in an appropriate way.

- Clearly he did understand what he was being asked to do. He was obviously trying to find the correct one-word name, and he did recognise that the answers that he had come up with were wrong. Even though losing the ability to reason is listed as a major early consequence of dementia, his response shows that this person was thinking about the question that he had been set.

- Although his answers were wrong, they were not random ones — they did have some connection with the word that he was looking for. Beavers aren't fish — but they do live in the water. Beavers are hairy creatures that look rather like large rats, even though they aren't rats. Certainly the one in the sketch the man was shown could have been mistaken for a rat!

- His comment about having seen this animal on television is perfectly reasonably, since this is the most likely place for someone who lives in Australia to have seen a beaver.

The links between the 'right' and 'wrong' names are discussed in more detail in chapter 5, where I outline strategies for making better sense of what someone with Alzheimer's is saying. Such links are very common in the naming errors of these people. Knowing this allows us to identify the core of good sense in much more confusing examples than this one.

Saying and doing something appropriate

As the beaver example shows, even when someone's dementia is well advanced, they are often capable of saying and doing something that is appropriate to the situation.

My mother, who had always been polite and well mannered, continued to be able to hold her own in casual social exchanges long after she was admitted to full-time care. She might not recognise the person who greeted her, but she would sense that they must be someone who knew her. *'How nice to see you'*, she would say, *'and how are the family?'* This — as my father noted — was a perfect response, since it applied to virtually everyone and gave visitors the impression that she still knew who they were.

> My mother also enjoyed being taken out to afternoon tea, and, again, even if she didn't always recognise the friends who had kindly invited us or the house where she had so often been before, she still knew how to behave on such occasions.

A number of the professional caregivers whom I met in France told me that they regularly and successfully take the people in their care on social outings.

Drawing on our memory for often-repeated words and actions

Although we commonly think of someone with Alzheimer's as having 'memory problems', it is useful to realise that 'memory' is actually made up of three different types and that these are affected differently by the dementing process. The ability to say and do what is appropriate to the occasion depends on what is known as **procedural memory.** This is our memory of activities or procedures that we have engaged in so often that they have become second nature to us. This type of memory survives much better and much longer in someone with dementia than do the other two types of memory — our memory for facts and figures (**semantic memory**) and our memory for the specific details of episodes in our own lives (**episodic memory**). Hence, even if someone has forgotten the date of an important national anniversary and forgotten how they celebrated it last year, they may still be able to enjoy celebrating it with us this year.

We draw on procedural memory when we engage in routine social exchanges, dance familiar dances, play familiar tunes on the piano, sing or recite well-known pieces, repeat the set of movements for performing a task that is a regular part of our work. All these are so deeply learnt that we perform them on auto-pilot as it were. Most people with dementia continue to be able to do these things if the circumstances are right; indeed sing-alongs and dance sessions are a regular activity in many residential homes and day-care centres.

> I remember with pleasure the sing-alongs at the home where my mother was. My mother would sing with gusto, usually producing the words of the first verse or chorus of well-known old songs with accuracy and improvising when she forgot. Growler would also join in,

jumping up and down on her lap. Her friend Wally, despite being unable to speak, could still help carry a tune by going *'dee-dee-dee'* and emphasising the beat with his arms. Even those residents who spent most of their time immobile and seemingly shrunk in on themselves would brighten up and start moving their bodies in time to the music.

The activities based on procedural memory are semi-automatic, but we shouldn't dismiss them as insignificant because of this. Even if an activity is semi-automatic it doesn't necessarily follow that the person is scarcely conscious of doing it, or that the activity has no value.

My mother was very much aware of her singing and social exchanges. She used to enjoy telling us about her performance during the singing sessions and the compliments that she received, making quite a story out of such incidents. Also she would often make some comment to me on the polite chitchat we had just exchanged with a fellow resident or visitor: *'I do think it's most important that one should thank people when they do kind things';* and *'I hope I got that right, Jane — it's important to be polite to people.'*

Sooner or later, though, even routine procedures will be slowed down or seriously interrupted by the dementing process. Getting dressed, going to the toilet, managing a knife and fork will become increasingly difficult to achieve. However, such is the resilience of procedural memory, that people with Alzheimer's can often be helped to maintain routines well beyond the stage when they start being disrupted, and can even, to a modest extent, learn new routines. What they depend upon is our providing the appropriate trigger to get the deeply learnt process underway again.

Triggers that helped my mother were the music and words of familiar songs at the regular sing-along sessions or the opening line of a favourite poem or nursery rhyme which we recited for her.

Such memories may explain otherwise bizarre behaviour

The survival of our memory of familiar procedures sometimes helps to explain behaviour that may well seem inappropriate and even bizarre.

A man in residential care in Melbourne was following the bed-making staff, removing the bedding from the bed they had just finished making, and tossing it up in the air. Once staff realised that he was keeping alive the routine gestures that he had used on sheep fleeces in his job as a wool-classer, they became much more sympathetic. He was provided with a suitable table and some old woollen blankets so that he could continue to practise an activity that was relevant to his sense of identity without disrupting the bed-makers.[v]

The crucial role of such memories when other means fail

The survival of our memory for often-repeated words and actions becomes even more crucial in the later stages of dementia.

In her last years my mother could still retrieve fragments of deeply imprinted items and use them to express herself when other means failed her. If she was lost for words she would resort to a familiar song — *'Oh what a beautiful morning'* always told us that she was enjoying herself. On one occasion I tried to jolly her out of a bad mood by singing this song myself, but she brought me up short by saying crossly, *'Don't sing that — it's not a proper song.'* Indeed, it was not a proper song to sing when she was feeling that the morning was far from beautiful. She would also adapt the words of such a song to help her say what she wanted — *'Oh what a beautiful daughter'* expressed her pleasure at a visit from me, *'Oh what a beautiful bear'* showed that she was enjoying a game with Growler.

In the final weeks and even days of her life she and my father kept in touch by means of familiar nursery rhymes — he would begin *'Sing a song of sixpence'* and she would echo his words and sometimes pick up the next line. This exchange may not seem very much, compared with the intelligent discussions they once shared, but it meant a great deal to my father because it told him that she was still aware of him as a friendly presence by her bedside.

Negative reactions may be appropriate too — in the circumstances

Many of the confused, angry or frightened reactions of people with dementia are also perfectly appropriate in the circumstances, as we realise if we consider what these circumstances actually are. Imagine that you are sitting or walking in a strange place — you don't know where you are and you feel quite sure that this is not where you should be — it isn't your home. A stranger comes up to you, grabs your arm and tries to get you to come with them. You would certainly feel alarmed and probably angry too; it would hardly be surprising if you thumped them. Yet such reactions by people with Alzheimer's are sometimes seen as irrational!

Similarly, you find yourself living in a place with a lot of other people and you vaguely remember that once you had a different sort of life. You wish that *'One day we might live somewhere on our own … Not in this sort of place where everyone lives.'* Most of the people except for your few favourites seem either *'quite mad'* or *'awfully dull … there's no one that's interesting at all. You think of them all. They're all as dull as dishwater.'* You sum up your impressions — *'When I'm here it feels like I'm nowhere'.* Despite the many admirable qualities of the residence where my mother was living and the pleasant times I knew she often had, I felt that her comments, which I have quoted here, were reasonable — even the best residence is not the same as your own home, and can be deadly boring at times.

'I'm terrified, I'm absolutely terrified … my one great terror is that the day will come when I feel that I ought to be doing something else and I forget what it is that I'm supposed to be doing … I'm sure to forget. I forget everything, I even forget when it's time to get up and when it's time to go to bed … I'm terrified of doing wrong … '

Comments like this are painful to listen to, but who wouldn't feel terrified being somewhere that feels strange and realising that your forgetfulness makes it that much harder to know what you are supposed to be doing; the experience is even more terrifying for someone like my mother who had been brought up to 'do the right thing'.

Dementing — but still able to think

Many of the examples that I have given so far suggest that someone with Alzheimer's is still capable of thinking. The idea that these people can and do still engage in what an ordinary person would call 'thinking' needs exploring further, given the fact that the loss of the ability to reason is widely recognised as a key early symptom of Alzheimer's disease. This, plus the implications of the term 'dementia' ('out of one's mind'), may well lead us to believe that anything worthy of being called 'thought' is beyond someone who is dementing. However, let's look more closely at what is involved in their losing the ability to reason.

- People who are dementing certainly have problems with their memory. Hence they will most probably be unable to summon up all the facts that we need to consider if we are to make an informed judgement or decision. (Retrieving facts and information depends on the semantic and episodic types of memory, which are the most seriously affected by dementia.)

- People with dementia lose the ability to distinguish between fact and fantasy. Real people they have met and events they have actually participated in get mixed up with people and events that they have simply imagined, read about or seen on television; in their memory, all now seem equally real. Past and present become similarly confused — people long dead and events long past may still seem part of their present reality. Hence the information that someone with dementia is working from may very well not be reliable.

- Because of their problems with short-term memory, they are likely to lose track of what they recently thought or did. This makes it difficult for them to 'think through' a question or to pick up their train of thought later. It also makes it very unlikely that they will still be able to form and carry out a detailed plan of action.

Because of all these factors, someone who is affected by Alzheimer's disease will certainly be unable to think as efficiently and productively as they once did. Inevitably they will lose the ability to manage their own affairs or look after their own material needs. However, being affected by the problems that I have just been describing is not quite the same thing as having no mind at all or being unable to think.

The point is worth insisting on, because if we believe that someone has 'lost their mind', we may well assume that everything that they say or do no longer makes sense and so cease trying to understand them. As 'Les' put it:

> Once you've got Alzheimer's you're branded. That was terrible. It still is terrible. I can't come to grips with that at all. It is so frustrating. Because I have Alzheimer's, what I say is irrelevant: nobody will listen.[vi]

Yet, as I hope this book helps to demonstrate, people like my mother and Les still have plenty to tell us if we are willing to listen to them.

Dementia interferes with effective reasoning but someone with the condition can still think about a situation and make deductions that are appropriate, given the circumstances. This point is illustrated by many of the explanations that my mother came up with for the situation in which she found herself. Because of the effects of her dementia these explanations were usually incorrect. However, they did make sense.

> She was not living at home and her husband was not living or sleeping with her. This is what had already happened during the war, so perhaps it was still wartime. She once tartly commented to me, *'What are husbands good for — just someone to write to!'* (This was a rare glimpse of the effort it must have been coping on her own during my father's long wartime absences, when she wrote to him every day.)
>
> Another explanation she came up with was that *'Tom must have lost all our money.'* Given that my father had always looked after our financial affairs, and that my mother's early memories would cover the period of the Great Depression this too seems a reasonable assumption for her to make.
>
> Similarly, since she didn't realise that she had dementia but was conscious of the fact that her leg was very sore, it was reasonable for her to assume that she was in hospital while recovering from an accident. This assumption was reinforced by the many hospital-like features of the residence where she was — nurses in uniform, corridors, hospital-like routines, people being cared for and some of them obviously very ill.
>
> Yet another, rather different example of appropriate thinking was her defence of an alteration she once made in her favourite nursery rhyme, *'Sing a song of sixpence'* . . . *'Along came a bulldog and pecked off her nose'.* When my father objected that the right word was 'blackbird', she replied: *'Yes, but a bulldog would be much more likely to peck off someone's nose!'*

Still able to feel and to express emotion

Even though people like my mother soon lose the ability to think accurately and productively about a situation, their capacity for feeling remains extremely strong. As some of the examples that I have already given demonstrate, my mother had plenty of feelings, both positive and negative, and was able to express them too. Indeed, people with dementia become less inhibited about expressing their feelings. This can sometimes be painful or embarrassing for those around them.

> My mother had occasional fits of misery, and she could be very outspoken about her dislike of one of the less sensitive members of the nursing staff — *'My word, she's a horror. I'd like to KILL her — and I will'.* The plus side was that when she seemed happy we knew that she really was happy since she no longer hid her feelings.

Even people in the final stages of dementia can still show their feelings.

> My mother used her deeply embedded memory of certain songs to express herself when she had trouble finding her own words.

Fortunately too, we can show our emotions without need for words — grunts, cries, hugs and movements can express emotions just as well. Carers who are alert to such signs will have the pleasure of recognising that they are still being responded to right up to the end.

A sense of humour

An important quality that makes us human is a sense of humour. This too is well known to survive in people with Alzheimer's disease.

> My mother continued to recognise jokes and to make jokes of her own. Once when I objected to going on an all-day car trip on the grounds that we might have problems finding a suitable toilet for her she said, with a chuckle, *'We could always go behind a hedge'.*
>
> The antics of the various cats and sparrows that hung around the home were a regular source of amusement to us both, as were many of the sayings and doings of Growler. My mother didn't only comment on Growler's activities, she also produced them — she even had a special growly voice that showed us when Growler was speaking or singing.
>
> My mother's sense of the difference between joking and being serious was clearly illustrated during an elaborate story she told me about

being invited to Buckingham Palace to eat a meal and see the treasures kept there. Whenever I made a frivolous suggestion, such as asking whether the treasures included any teddy bears, she would laugh and join in the joke; then she would return to her story by saying *'I really mean this Jane'* or *'But seriously, Jane'.* I found it intriguing that this joking/being serious distinction still held for her, despite the fact that she had by now lost the ability to distinguish fact from fantasy — as the mixture of ingredients that made up her Buckingham Palace story showed.

SUMMING UP — THE ABILITIES NEEDED FOR KEEPING IN TOUCH

Despite the effects of dementia someone with Alzheimer's will usually be capable of:

- interacting with another person;

- responding appropriately to a situation;

- thinking about something;

- repeating deeply learnt words, movements and gestures;

- feeling and expressing emotion;

- expressing ideas;

- being aware of and reflecting on something that they have done;

- making and responding to jokes;

- telling stories.

It is indeed possible to keep in touch with someone who has Alzheimer's. Despite the problems caused by their condition, they still have the basic abilities that are involved in making contact with and responding to other people.

My mother continued to be good at routine social exchanges and was aware of their value. She established and maintained contact with some of the nursing staff after she was in full-time professional care and developed a special friendship with another resident. She also continued to respond to my father's and my attempts at maintaining our previously close relationships with her.

Specialists in communication believe that making and maintaining contact with others is a key function of language and communication.[vii] A large proportion of the communicating that all of us do is basically about keeping in touch. Routine greetings, a smile and a wave, a chat about nothing much, a friendly phone call or postcard, a quick e-mail — these keep us in social contact with other members of our community. The content of these social exchanges is relatively unimportant; what counts is their role in binding us together and giving us our sense of belonging. Positive contact with others is essential for maintaining our sense of identity and worth and this is especially true for someone with Alzheimer's.

CHAPTER 2

RECOGNISING AND ALLOWING FOR THE PROBLEMS THAT WILL OCCUR

WHAT THIS CHAPTER COVERS

Even though I don't want to place too much emphasis on the negative side of the picture, it does help to know something about the difficulties that Alzheimer's disease usually causes. This helps us in two ways:

- *It prevents us blaming people with the condition for problems that are beyond their control.*

- *It tells us what allowances we may need to make when interacting with them.*

Before covering the various types of problem in roughly the order in which they are likely to occur, though, I consider the question of the general nature of these problems. Is it a matter of memories and capacities being lost, or do these simply become increasingly hard to get access to?

At the end of this chapter I stress two important points that we need to keep in mind when we are considering the problems associated with Alzheimer's disease:

- *Our own reactions may sometimes contribute to the problems that we may be experiencing.*

- *We need to guard against jumping to conclusions and underestimating what someone with Alzheimer's is saying or doing. I illustrate this by two real-life examples in which someone with Alzheimer's showed more ability than they had been given credit for.*

LOST? OR JUST BECOMING HARDER TO FIND?

Before considering the problems that someone with Alzheimer's is likely to have with memory and words, it is interesting to know that there is some uncertainty about the exact nature of these problems. Has the person with

23

dementia actually lost the memories and words in question, as we tend to imagine? Or are they simply having problems getting access to them?

- That the problem may often be one of access rather than loss is suggested by the fact that these people often have good days, when they can do and remember things that they couldn't the day before.

- Another significant fact is that people with dementia tend to score better on tests if they are given much more time to come up with the answers.

- Plenty of mental structures, processes and associations do survive the alterations produced by dementia.

To put it more simply, the mistakes that people with Alzheimer's make are not as random as they might be if the contents of their mind had simply fallen apart. Instead, the mistakes are like what happens when we go to a familiar store-cupboard or bookshelf in the dark — we reach in to grab the item that we want but, instead, we may well end up with the item stored next to it.

PROBLEMS THAT THEY ARE LIKELY TO HAVE

The problems below are given in roughly the order in which they are likely to start occurring in someone with Alzheimer's. I am concentrating on those problems which interfere the most with understanding and keeping in touch (such as problems with memory and language), and will mention other, more physical problems only as they contribute to these.

Lapses of memory

One of the first symptoms of Alzheimer's disease is lapses of memory.

> My mother started forgetting what she had done yesterday or what we had planned for today. She would forget that she had just had breakfast, and be cross at my father (who used to bring her breakfast in bed) for the apparent delay.

Such lapses of memory are not necessarily a sign of the early stages of dementia. Most people have slips of this sort from time to time. However, it becomes obvious that something may be wrong when memory lapses become more and more frequent.

> My mother's forgetfulness gradually reached a point where she was finding it hard to keep track of whatever she was doing. She was no longer able to cook, make clothes, look after her favourite rockeries or even read a book. These are extended activities that depend on our remembering what we have already done or read and where we are in the process, as well as knowing what we need to do next. My mother would start the same book over and over, without realising it. Moreover, we could no longer leave her on her own, since she would forget where we were or what was going on and would rapidly become distressed by our absence. But because of her procedural memory there were plenty of routine pleasures that my mother could still enjoy. With us to help her out as necessary, she was able to live at home and lead a fairly normal life for a number of years. Few visitors would have realised that she had Alzheimer's.

In the earlier stages of dementia it is fairly easy for family and friends to compensate for forgetfulness by tactful reminders: *'I so enjoyed our drive around the lake yesterday'*; *'I'm looking forward to John's visit this evening.'* Care centres and residential homes often run a program of what is called 'reality orientation' to provide systematic reminders of basic information — the date, time of year, key anniversaries and current events — to help people with dementia retain their orientation to the here and now.

When memory problems become really serious, though, these systematic attempts to help someone keep track become counterproductive. They simply rub in the fact that this person can't remember things properly any more. At this stage we can help them more by concentrating on such immediately relevant information as where the toilets are or where their bedroom is. Simple strategies like leaving the door open so that the toilet is visible, for instance, can help here.

Moods

Most people are able to control their moods to suit the circumstances. We can usually manage to put on a smiling face in public, even though we may be feeling unhappy or unwell. However, people with dementia tend to show what they are really feeling. Moreover, the mood that they are in at a given moment will colour everything around them.

> When my mother was feeling happy, everything pleased her. If she was feeling cross, though, it was a different matter. She would point accusingly at a garden that she had praised extravagantly yesterday and shout *'appalling, that's appalling'*.

Realising that the responses of a person with dementia often reflect their inner mood helps one to understand apparently inconsistent reactions of this sort to their external environment.

Problems finding the right name

Another common symptom of dementia is having trouble giving people and items their correct name. A standard test for dementia is based on this. However, this problem doesn't mean that someone with Alzheimer's starts talking nonsense. The example in the previous chapter of how one person responded to the test picture of a beaver shows just how relevant what they say can be, even if they can't find the word that they are looking for. Recognising how the wrong name and the right one are related is a key strategy for understanding what they are saying.

> My mother had a number of perfectly good ways of referring to her favourite fruit, bananas, even if she couldn't recall their exact name. Similarly, her calling animals that she liked *'bears'* ceased to be simply a mistake if you knew that what she meant by this was *'cuddly, furry animals like my bear Growler'*.

Misnaming members of one's family is another example of this symptom, and one that often upsets carers. However, this too is usually meaningful, showing recognition of the sort of person that we are.

In the early stages of dementia any such naming difficulties are hardly a problem, since the person will ask us for the right name, or will come up with an alternative way of saying what they want to, such as *'that fruit I like to eat'*. In the later stages, when their store of available words has become smaller, they may cope as my mother did when she couldn't remember the word 'mountain' by pointing and saying *that thing over there'*. However, the cumulative effect of the various problems that develop in their use of words may make it increasing difficult for us to interpret what they are saying.

Repeating themselves

Caregivers often find it very irritating when the person with Alzheimer's asks the same question over and over again. However, because of their problems with remembering recent events, they most probably don't realise that they have already asked the question and that it has been answered. Knowing this encourages us to be more patient in our responses.

Repeated questions may sometimes be an implicit appeal for attention and reassurance, as Frena Gray-Davidson points out in her book for carers.[viii] Bear in mind that someone with Alzheimer's has good reason to feel worried and insecure. Ignoring their questions or giving an impatient response just makes the problem worse. Instead we need to identify the anxiety that underlies the question and spend some time addressing that.

As their dementia progresses, people become increasingly likely to repeat themselves. They seem to get stuck in a groove, as it were.

> My mother could keep going on endless variations of one of her favourite stories for a whole morning, and would be more than happy to sing the same song over and over. Again, this can easily be very irritating, but I coped by reminding myself that my mother had trouble remembering these things. Hence, when a story or a song did come to mind this was a real achievement for her; and, once she got started, it was much easier and more satisfying for her to continue than to find something fresh to say.

Mixing past and present events

As recent events become harder to remember, past ones tend to become more vivid.

> In the early stages of her dementia my mother enjoyed retelling us stories about her childhood; her ability to recall details of the distant past helped to compensate for her increasing fits of forgetfulness about what was happening in the present.

Gradually, though, the distinction between past and present disappears and people and happenings long past become part of the present reality of someone with Alzheimer's. Hence we can often make better sense of what they are saying or doing if we relate it to what we know of their past life.

> When my mother talked about having moved the rocks around in the hospital garden, this was untrue, but we realised that she was reliving gardening activities from years ago. Rather than correcting her, we would enter into the spirit of what she was saying and praise her skills as a gardener.

> The past was also still very much alive for Stavros, a resident of a nursing home who started pulling up tomato seedlings as fast as the gardener and other residents planted them. When the Director of Nursing asked why, he replied, *'Because when they are ripe, the Turks will come along and steal them and there will not be any for us.'* This was hardly likely to happen in Australia, where Stavros had now lived for many years, it but would have been a real threat in his homeland. The Director reassured Stavros by entering into his reality and promising him that if the Turks came, she would *'fight them off'*. [ix]

Fact and fantasy become equally real

Sometimes we have trouble distinguishing between something we have actually done and something we have merely thought about — 'Did I remember to turn off the oven, or did I just think about doing it?' Most of the time, though, we know perfectly well what is fact and what is just something we have read or dreamt about or seen on television.

Someone with Alzheimer's, though, loses the ability to separate fact from fantasy. Everything that comes into their minds seems equally real to them. Once this happens, it is unfair to think of them as lying to us when they tell us something that we know isn't true. Tact is necessary here — if they are making claims that are obviously important to them, it is kinder to accept their reality than to contradict them.

> My mother was perfectly happy for us to tell her that the tea trolley hadn't come by yet, but doubting the stories she told us about herself was another matter. *'Are you calling me a liar?'* she demanded angrily on one occasion when my father was looking sceptical about her account of diving for treasure in the lake. The story was clearly untrue. Quite apart from the fantastic details about the treasure itself, my mother had never been a good swimmer and had not swum in the lake for years.

The important point about this story was not whether it was true or untrue, but the fact that it helped my mother feel strong and capable at a time when her dementia was making her increasingly helpless. Recognising the psychological function helped us to be supportive of the need being expressed rather than rejecting the stories out of hand because they were untrue.

Another important point to keep in mind is that losing the ability to distinguish fact from fantasy doesn't mean that everything that someone with Alzheimer's tells us is untrue. Some of my mother's stories were indeed substantially true, and others had a solid grain of truth in them — as did her gardening claims and Stavros's fears that the Turks would take the tomatoes. Moreover, someone with Alzheimer's is extremely vulnerable to being tricked or exploited by other people. Hence it would be unwise to dismiss every account of having been robbed or otherwise harmed as merely a delusion produced by dementia. In some instances, they may be right. Even if they are wrong, we should respond sympathetically since we know about the memory and other problems that are causing them to make such claims.

Telling fantastic stories about themselves

The loss of the ability to distinguish fact from fantasy is most strikingly demonstrated in the stories that people with Alzheimer's tell us about themselves.

> My mother's obviously untrue account of diving for treasure in the local lake is one example of such a story. Another, even more fantastic example, is her claim to have slain vast numbers of enemy soldiers on the top of the nearby mountain: *'I bounced out at them . . . BASH, BASH, BASH . . . Do you know how many I counted up when I removed*

all the corpses? I counted up that I had made 37 000!' Perhaps not surprisingly, this exploit earns her the Victoria Cross and *'a lot of other very precious medals'*.

In the medical literature on dementia such stories are referred to as **pseudo-reminiscence** or **confabulation.** Because of their indiscriminate mixture of true and fantastic elements and the way they get endlessly repeated, such stories may seem very confused. However, they have considerable value for their teller.

Seeing things

Some people with dementia start 'seeing things'. They talk to invisible people or pets, or are frightened of something that no-one else can see or hear. As well as having hallucinations of this sort, they may also misinterpret some element of their environment. For example, they may refuse to step onto a shiny patch of floor, or to cross the join between two colours of carpet or linoleum because they interpret the difference as meaning there is a deep puddle or a hole in front of them. They may also talk to their reflection in the mirror. The fact that they have forgotten what they now look like contributes to the illusion that their reflection is another person.

Sometimes such hallucinations or mistaken interpretations are a source of pleasure, in which case it makes sense to accept them. If they are causing distress, we can provide a positive distraction or remove the stimulus that is producing them — by shifting or doing away with the mirror, for instance, if the old person in it seems menacing rather than friendly.

In some cases, though, misinterpretation may simply be an effect of failing eyesight or hearing rather than of dementia.

My mother sometimes mistook a windblown leaf for a bird — but I could see the 'bird' too if I simply took off my glasses.

Echoing what is said to them

As access to words becomes more difficult and their vocabulary shrinks, people with Alzheimer's are sometimes reduced to doing little more than echoing what is said to them. However, even this minimal response tells us that they have heard us and are responding as best they can. Rather than seeing such echoing as mere parroting, we need to value it as a surviving means of interaction — a way of still being in touch with us.

Speaking in fragments

Problems with 'finding the right words' also result in people with Alzheimer's speaking in fragments rather than full sentences. Strategies that we can use to fill such fragments out and understand them better are given in chapter 5.

Being not here but somewhere else

People with Alzheimer's have periods of seeming to be somewhere else — of having what, in a normal person, we might call a fit of daydreaming or abstraction. Maybe they are 'tuning out' or 'switching off' for a while from the effort involved in remembering things and keeping their world together. Maybe they are indeed somewhere else, just as we are when we daydream.

If they seem calm and contented, there is no point in disrupting them unless there is a good reason. In the later stages of dementia however some people do seem to become increasingly turned in on themselves and detached from what is happening around them. Attempts to keep in touch with them can prevent this happening unduly or make it less frequent. Sometimes though, and especially towards the end, some people with dementia may not respond to such attempts any more, and often carers prefer to let them be, seeing this as part of the withdrawal that can be a prelude to death. Other people with Alzheimer's may be responsive to us even in the final days of their life, as my mother was. However withdrawn someone with dementia may seem, being there in case they need us is certainly worthwhile.

Increasing physical problems

Physical difficulties may also add to the problems that I've been describing. Sometimes the person has existing handicaps, like the sciatica and deteriorating hip joints that were already giving my mother trouble with walking before the onset of Alzheimer's. Then the dementing process itself sooner or later interferes with the ability to perform physical tasks unaided. Eating, moving about, dressing, washing, going to the toilet — everything becomes progressively harder. Although it is possible to help someone with dementia retain these functions longer than is sometimes realised, sooner or later they do become a major problem.

I will not be discussing these physical problems in detail, since ways of dealing with them are given in a number of other books for carers which are available from support groups such as the Alzheimer's Association. However, the strategies for keeping in touch, which are my concern here, should help you interact more positively with someone with dementia while you are helping them with daily care.

FACTORS THAT MAY BE ADDING UNNECESSARILY TO THE PROBLEM

Because someone has dementia there is always the risk that we may overlook or dismiss problems that are not directly caused by dementia but which are making its symptoms seem worse than they really are.

Eyesight

Some misnamings or other confusions may simply be due to poor eyesight — or dirty spectacles!

> When my mother thought a windblown leaf was a small bird, this was not a hallucination produced by her dementia but the result of not being able to see properly. If I took off my glasses, or screwed up my eyes I could see that it looked like a bird too. I learned always to check that she was wearing the right glasses (and that they were clean!) before we did anything together.

Hearing

Hearing problems can add to communication difficulties. If the person wears a hearing aid, it still needs to be switched on and have a battery that functions. If the person does have hearing problems, conversation will be more pleasant with them in a quiet and less distracting setting — this makes it much easier for both people to concentrate. Speak clearly (not loudly), look at the person so that they can see your facial expression and the movement of your lips, and don't be afraid to repeat yourself. These strategies will help you communicate with someone with dementia whether they have hearing problems or not.

Effects of medication

If someone with Alzheimer's is slow to respond to you, this may be due to drugs that they are being given to manage their condition. Check what medication is being given, and don't hesitate to make your views known if you feel that the person you care about is being adversely affected. You may not be a medical expert but you are an expert on this person and on what helps or hinders interaction between you both.

Recently there has been a definite move away from using drugs to control someone with dementia. Indeed, many professional carers now believe that it is morally wrong to use a treatment that will slow down even further the mental and physical responses of someone affected by dementia. If you are looking for suitable residential care for someone with dementia, check out the institution's policy on medications. Lots of dopey-looking people slumped in chairs is a bad sign — not of their dementia but of the lack of a positive care program. Unfortunately, in some places, chemical and physical restraints are still routinely used — it is less bother to cope with troublesome patients by giving them a pill and strapping them into a chair than trying to supply the activities and supportive environment that might prevent their being troublesome in the first place.

Depression

Many of the early symptoms of dementia are very similar to those of depression — so much so that textbooks warn health professionals of the possibility of confusing the two conditions. Hence it is important to have a formal diagnosis made before you jump to the conclusion that someone's forgetfulness and confusion are due to Alzheimer's. Even if they do have Alzheimer's, they may also be depressed and this will aggravate their symptoms. Indeed, if they realise that they have something seriously wrong with them or have registered that they have dementia, they have good reason to feel depressed.

Periodic bouts of unhappiness or worry are part of being human. People with Alzheimer's have them like anyone else. However, if these are occurring too often and lasting too long, we may be looking at depression as well as dementia. Pleasant stimulus and friendly, supportive interaction with others helps both conditions.

Boredom and frustration

I have added boredom and frustration to this checklist because many of the problem behaviours associated with Alzheimer's are caused by these. As someone finds it more difficult to initiate and carry out many of the tasks or hobbies that used to keep them busy and amused, they become more dependent on people helping them to engage in suitable activities.

Better specialised care units have a full program of activities to suit the needs of even severely demented residents and so make their day interesting. People with Alzheimer's are also dependent on our goodwill in making it possible for them to engage in activities they have chosen for themselves, such as wandering about.

> My mother had always enjoyed pottering about out of doors, and became very frustrated if she couldn't do this. She was much happier if she had a safe space where she could wander or a supportive person to accompany her.

One of the most pleasant ways of passing the time though, is being with someone who shows that they care for you enough to want to spend time with you.

WHO IS HAVING THE PROBLEM — THEM OR US?

To conclude this list of problems, it is worth considering whether the real problem is the other person's dementia or our reaction to it. Our negative feelings about dementia may make us reluctant to spend time with someone who has the condition and unwilling to give them our full attention when we do. Or our consciousness of what they can't do, and the things we can no longer do together, may prevent us accepting and enjoying being with the person that they are now. This is why this book pays most attention to the more positive side of the picture — not what has been lost but what remains, what these people can still do, and what we can do to keep in touch with them.

DON'T UNDERESTIMATE SOMEONE WITH DEMENTIA!

Even though frequently we have to allow for the problems caused by Alzheimer's disease, we need to guard against underestimating the person with the condition. Because we know they have dementia it is easy to assume the worst and to interpret something that they say or do as a symptom of their dementia rather than checking whether it has some other significance in its own right. The following two incidents illustrate what I mean.

My mother remembers

The first incident occurred when my mother had already been some time in residential care.

'What's that name I used to call you?' she asked me suddenly.

'Jane,' I replied, jumping to the conclusion that she'd already forgotten my name and trying to conceal my dismay.

'I know that,' she said in disgusted tones. *'What's that other name I used to call you?'*

Then I realised what she meant — as I should have done had I been paying proper attention to her words. She hadn't said, *'What's your name?'* but was asking about a name that she 'used to call' me. She was seeking my help in recalling a private piece of affectionate by-play that we had often indulged in, dating back to the time when we had a farm.

'Your little ewe lamb,' I replied.

'That's right! Baaaah!'

'Meeeh!' And we started to mimic a ewe calling her lamb and the lamb's reply.

(The term 'ewe lamb' for a beloved only daughter comes from the Victorian novels that we had enjoyed together; we not only used this term but improved on it by imitating the noises we had heard our own sheep make.)

Eventually my mother did have some trouble recalling my name but that was still some years in the future. Moreover, forgetting someone's name doesn't necessarily mean losing all sense of who they are. I was happy to be identified by my mother during my last visit to her as *'a very important person'.*

The patient who was not as dumb as she seemed

My other incident comes from Mitra Khosravi, a psychologist and physiotherapist who works in Paris with people who have Alzheimer's disease. As she writes in her book for carers:

> I was witness to the following scene:
>
> A well-known professor was applying some clinical tests to a female patient to determine how advanced her dementia was. He ordered her to *'lift the left hand', 'shake the right leg', 'give my hand a good squeeze'* etc. But he got no response. Instead, the patient became agitated and made us understand that she wanted to go to the toilet. Once there, much to my amazement she confided to me, *'He really irritates me, that stupid bearded chap with his silly questions. I'll stay here so that he gets irritated and pushes off!'* Incidentally, this woman patient had always disliked bearded men!
>
> This incident taught me my lesson, and I promised myself that in the future I would be less hasty in judging the silence or failure to respond of someone with Alzheimer's.[x]

CHAPTER 3

MAKING THE MOST OF BEING TOGETHER

WHAT THIS CHAPTER COVERS

This chapter covers a range of strategies for ensuring that your interactions with the person for whom you care go as well as possible. They include details of:

- *how to approach the other person*

- *what sort of setting is most appropriate*

- *the role of nonverbal signals and of touch*

- *how pets and soft toys may provide a useful stimulus for some people.*

GETTING OFF TO A GOOD START

First impressions count

Interactions with someone who has Alzheimer's will have a better chance of succeeding if you get off to a good start. I am thinking in particular of someone who is sufficiently advanced in the dementing process that we have to take their condition into account when we approach them. They may well be living in a specialised residence by this stage.

Even though my mother would sometimes be vaguely expecting me to appear, thanks to the friendly prompts and comments of the staff about my coming to visit her, I knew that I shouldn't rush things. I kept in mind that someone with Alzheimer's often needs extra time for something to register properly. Hence, whenever possible, I gave her sufficient time to realise that someone was coming towards her — someone who obviously knew and liked her. I would approach her from the front, waving while still at a distance to attract her attention, and showing by my broad smile and relaxed and friendly manner that I was really pleased to see her. By the time I reached her, she was usually already responding and eager for the hug and kiss that was our standard form of greeting. Our special family friend Olwen, who visited my mother regularly right up to the end of her life, used the same approach.

What we did, in fact, was continue to approach my mother as we had always done but taking care to give her time to recognise what was happening. Even when she finally had trouble recalling our exact relationship to her — beloved daughter, old friend — she still recognised that she was being greeted lovingly by someone close to her and would respond accordingly. Our body language was obviously a crucial ingredient in our approach.

As well as helping my mother, this slower approach also gave us time to assess her mood. Her body language would alert us to whether she was contented, bored, abstracted or agitated and we could take this into account in our opening remarks.

If you are visiting someone regularly you may find it helpful to develop and stick to some form of opening ritual.

My father, on his daily visit to my mother when she was in residential care, always brought her a piece of fresh fruit. This provided a ready-made basis for interaction and conversation between them. This ritual had the added advantage of being reassuringly familiar to my mother.

Because memory for often-repeated routines tends to survive reasonably well, doing what we have done many times before is easier than doing something different, especially if we have Alzheimer's.

The value of getting off to a good start becomes very apparent if you watch what happens during the visits other residents are receiving. Some people are clearly awkward and embarrassed in the presence of a person who has Alzheimer's. They introduce themselves too abruptly and they make it immediately obvious by their stiffness and their forced cheerfulness that they would rather be somewhere else. The visit may be well-intentioned, but it gives no pleasure to anyone.

- *Give the other person time to register your presence*

- *Show that you are pleased to see them*

Dealing with a hostile reception

Even if your visits are usually a success, at times the person you care for may be unresponsive or hostile towards you. I was fortunate in that this rarely happened to me, but when it did I learnt that it was better to leave my mother for a while and try again later.

There are three good reasons for doing this.

1. If we become tense and agitated ourselves the situation can only get worse, since people with Alzheimer's are very responsive to our moods.

2. We may unwittingly be the cause of their hostile reactions.

> Occasionally when my father visited her, my mother would become fixed on the difference between an earlier time when they were living and sleeping together and the present. The longer he stayed, the angrier she would become. My father soon found that, if his efforts to make the visit more pleasant were having no effect, it was kinder to both of them simply to go away. If he returned half an hour later, she would usually have forgotten her earlier anger and be delighted to see him.

3. There is no point in exhausting yourself unnecessarily by staying around when things are not going well. It is much better to retreat and give yourself time to recover your spirits before trying again.

- *If a hostile response persists, retreat and try again later*

CHOOSING AN APPROPRIATE SETTING

The setting itself can contribute to the success or failure of our interactions with someone who has Alzheimer's. A basic rule is that a peaceful, familiar setting with no distractions makes it easier for both of you to relax and to give each other your full attention. Keep in mind that someone with Alzheimer's usually finds it easier to cope with one thing at a time. If there is something interesting going on, such as an organised activity or the impromptu entertainment provided by a visitor with a small dog or by a cleaner sweeping the floor, use this as the focus of your interaction. Enjoy it together; make it the topic of your conversation. If the distraction is a potentially disturbing one, it makes sense to find a more tranquil spot for the two of you.

> My mother didn't care for loud noises or overly boisterous children.

Seating that lets you be close together is an advantage too.

> The home where my mother was had a number of two-person settees in which we could sit together very companionably. Because these were made of cane they were light and easy to move, so I was able to choose an appropriate position for us within the room — facing the garden, for instance. When my mother was in her wheelchair, I would draw up a chair for myself beside or at right angles to her so that it was easy for us to see and touch each other, to play together with Growler or to look at a magazine.

Some settings go with certain regular activities — eating together in the dining room, sorting out clothes in the bedroom, joining the group around the piano for the regular sing-along session. Such settings reinforce the activity that takes place in them and make it easier for someone with Alzheimer's to participate appropriately, especially if their dementia is at all advanced.

Other settings may be associated with special pleasures.

> My mother especially enjoyed going out into the garden with us. Formerly a keen gardener, she still liked being out of doors and among plants. Some of our best times together were spent in the garden. She and I had our favourite spot too — an out-of-the-way corner where we could sing loudly together without disturbing other people.
>
> Another treat was being driven to a lakeside park where she could throw bread to the seagulls.

> - *Peaceful, familiar settings help you to relax together*
>
> - *One distraction at a time is enough*
>
> - *Interaction is easier if you are close together*
>
> - *Specific settings reinforce the activity that routinely happens there*

BEING AWARE OF NONVERBAL SIGNALS

Getting off to a good start depends upon being aware of and exploiting nonverbal signals. Our body language as we approach someone tells them that we are a friend coming to visit them. Similarly, their body language alerts us to their current mood and also lets us know whether they have registered our approach and welcome it.

Because of the problems people with Alzheimer's frequently have in expressing themselves via words, all the nonverbal aspects of communication become increasingly important. If you know someone well, they can communicate a great deal to you without a word being spoken. Their face, especially their eyes and the set of their mouth, their gestures, how they hold themselves, how they move, all convey their mood. Because I had always been close to my mother I was already conscious of her body language, but I made an effort to become even more aware of it, knowing the help that this would give me in the later stages of her dementia.

The following incident brought home to me the important role that our body language — in this case my own — can play in our interactions with the person for whom we care.

> At the start of one of my visits my mother was sitting in a low chair. As I approached she looked up at me and exclaimed, *'Oh, Jane — how tall you've grown!'* Immediately I dropped down on my knees, and asked, *'Is this better?'* *'Yes, much better!'* she replied.

My mother's strongest memories of me were as I was when a child. Having me tower over her was confusing, whereas if I made myself smaller than her this reinforced our old relationship of mother and child. I kept this in mind during all subsequent interactions with her, deliberately choosing a lower chair for myself, for example, or snuggling down and putting my head on her shoulder when we were together in the two-seater settee. (Fortunately, my mother was much taller than I am, so keeping myself the appropriate size for a daughter was fairly easy.)

Noticing a range of nonverbal signals

A simple strategy for alerting yourself to the range of nonverbal signals that communicate our feelings to others is to stand in front of a mirror and deliberately act out various emotions. The following list will help you to notice some of the key signals that we give.

• **Eyes**: Note what your eyelids and eyebrows do, depending on whether you are alert, sleepy, puzzled, alarmed etc. (Keep in mind that medication may produce a drowsy look — if the person that you care for often seems drowsy or is drowsy at inconvenient times, check whether they are being over-sedated.)

• **Mouth**: Smile, look sad, look surprised, look disapproving. Note how your mouth turns up or down depending on your mood, and how the lines around your mouth act as reinforcement. (Older people sometimes develop lines that make them look more glum than they may feel — it helps to know what their normal, at rest expression is, so that you can spot any changes from this.) Your mouth and chin may well tremble if you are feeling truly miserable — my mother's did.

• **Gestures**: Most of us have a range of fairly routine gestures which we use to emphasise our words.

> '*That's appalling,*' my mother would exclaim, and point her arm accusingly at whatever it was that was offending her. '*It happened there,*' she would say during one of her stories about herself, gesturing towards the mountain or lake or shop where the events were supposed to have happened.

However, many gestures communicate without the help of words. You see someone you love coming towards you — note how your arms prepare for the hug you are going to greet them with. Someone you dislike or feel angry towards? You may well fold your arms in a certain way, or, if you are uninhibited or sufficiently outraged, you may shake your fist or give them the finger! (Professional carers need to be alert to cultural differences here. Some communities have a highly developed and specific set of meaningful gestures, and woe betide the outsider who unwittingly produces the wrong gesture at the wrong time.)

- **Stance and movement**: How you hold yourself and move also communicate a great deal. I've already mentioned my mother's reaction to the fact that I seemed unnaturally tall for her daughter, and how I tried to reinforce our relationship by taking up positions that kept me 'smaller' than her. On an everyday basis, our moods are communicated to others by our stance and movement. Note how your whole body becomes alert when you are interested in something, and how it droops if you are feeling exhausted or sad. If you are contented, you relax; if you are agitated you may well pace up and down.

> My mother liked to be up and moving about — my father and I could readily tell the difference between comfortable pottering and restless agitation.

- **Tone of voice**: When we speak, part of our meaning is conveyed by our tone of voice. Hence, even if you don't understand someone's words, you often get a general impression of what they are trying to say. Again, you can alert yourself to this aspect of communication by deliberately changing your voice and noticing how this changes the implications of what you are saying. *'You silly thing,'* for example, can be said in an angry or accusing tone of voice, in a resigned tone, or in an affectionate tone. *'What?'* is not only a question — it can also express amazement, disbelief or disgust, depending on how we say it. My mother's *'What'* meant all of these on different occasions.

Other indications of how we feel about what we are saying include how loudly we speak, how rapidly, how emphatically, and whether our voice is firm or shaky.

> The voice in which my mother told me a story about something she had achieved was emphatic and confident. The voice in which she expressed her fears was more reedy and quavering. When Growler was supposed to be speaking my mother used an appropriately growly tone of voice.

> - *Tone of voice and body language reveal our feelings*
>
> - *Learn to read these signals in the person for whom you care*

Be aware of the signals you send

All these nonverbal signals help us to understand the person with Alzheimer's. However, don't forget that we are sending the same sort of signals to them, too. Carers across the world agree that people with Alzheimer's are extremely sensitive to the body language of others. It is essential to be aware of this if we want to communicate positively with them. There is no point in saying something pleasant if our tone of voice and stiffness of body make it all too clear that we are nervous about, or even actively dislike being in contact with, someone who has dementia. Similarly, forced cheerfulness or false heartiness won't necessarily mask the feelings that we may be trying to hide.

> My mother was quick at spotting whether we accepted or doubted her stories. *'Are you calling me a liar?'* she demanded angrily of my father on one occasion. (Even though he had said nothing, she had noticed his raised eyebrows.) Even when her dementia was well advanced, her reactions showed me that she was still able to distinguish the genuine friendliness of the woman who took around the trolley for morning and afternoon tea from the laboured cheerfulness of a less-than-sympathetic member of staff.

I cannot pretend that I never felt reluctant or nervous about encountering my mother during the period when she was increasingly affected by dementia. However, I developed a personal routine of pushing such feelings aside and concentrating on the essential purpose of my visit — giving her pleasure and showing her that I still cared about her. It helped to think of this in physical terms — at a particular point when I entered the hospital grounds, I 'magicked' myself back into my well-established role as her beloved daughter and loving friend. I also took my own advice, and took my leave if my presence became unwelcome, and tried again later.

> - *Be alert to what your body language is telling them too*

TOUCH — A SPECIAL MEANS OF COMMUNICATION

One of the reasons for calling this book 'keeping in touch' is the importance of touch in the literal sense in our contacts with someone for whom we care.

Touch is a way of showing our affection for someone. We hug them when we meet, and hold their hand or arm when talking or walking together.

> My mother and I had always been physically demonstrative towards each other, and this habit helped me to maintain a close relationship with her.

Even if someone hasn't been particularly demonstrative in the past, they may well become more so as their dementia develops. People with Alzheimer's often lose their earlier inhibitions about expressing their feelings openly. Also they seem to have a greater need for the reassurance that affectionate physical contact provides. Indeed, this is a very basic need that dates from our infancy, when touch was all-important in our relationship with our first caregiver.

Touch can also contribute to our interactions with someone with Alzheimer's. When we are listening or talking to them, holding their hand or arm is a way of showing our interest and getting their attention.

> When my mother was in an advanced stage of dementia my father spent a lot of time reciting nursery rhymes with her. While they did this, he would hold her hands and move them in time to the rhythm of the words.

Grooming is another means of physical contact with someone. Simple activities like hair-brushing, giving a manicure, or rubbing in hand cream are a pleasant and relaxing way of passing the time. Applying hand-cream provides an acceptable form of contact for someone who isn't used to being demonstrative in public, as my father discovered when my mother was moved into full-time care.

You can also ask the other person to touch you.

> My mother was pleased to be asked to rub my back.

As the other person comes to need more help with their normal daily activities, this will involve us in physical contact with them too. Do as you would be done by here — warm hands, and a firm but considerate touch are much more agreeable than being handled as if you are a senseless slab of meat! Bear in mind though that help with bathing or showering, going to the toilet, and possibly dressing, are often better left to professional carers. Not only do they know the proper way to do these things without straining their own backs unduly, but often the person who needs help with more intimate matters prefers this to be done by someone who isn't a family member. I was willing enough to help my mother in the earlier stages of her dementia, but once she was in full-time care and needed considerably more help than formerly I was happy to leave this side of things to others and save my energies for more interesting activities with her. Bearing in mind how readily someone with Alzheimer's picks up on our body language, it is certainly unwise to assist with bathing or toileting if you feel at all uneasy or embarrassed about doing so.

- *Touch is a simple way of expressing affection*

- *Simple everyday activities involve touch, like grooming*

- *Some aspects of physical help may be best left to professional carers*

PETS AND TOYS AS A POSSIBLE FOCUS FOR INTERACTION

Their advantages

For many people with Alzheimer's, pets or soft toys are an invaluable resource.

> My mother never ceased to take pleasure in animals and in her teddy bear, Growler.

As well as giving pleasure, pets or soft toys serve two other extremely important functions.

- They help to keep the attention of the person with dementia turned outwards towards their environment, thus counteracting the tendency to turn more and more inwards on themselves.

- They provide a ready-made topic of conversation and focus for interaction with others. After all, unless you know the other person or have previous experience of someone with dementia, it can be hard to think of what on earth to say to them.

> A great number of the exchanges between passers-by and my mother centred on Growler; without this obvious source of comment, she would probably have been ignored on many occasions.

Pets don't worry about the fact that someone has dementia. For a cat, a warm lap is a warm lap.

Pets provide opportunities for exercise — playing with a cat or taking a dog for a walk are simple, satisfying activities.

A pet is an additional responsibility for carers, but one that may well repay the effort. Many residential homes have their resident cat or dog.

> My parents' cat sometimes accompanied my father on his visits, and I have seen the whole room brighten up when she appeared — especially if she co-operated by playing with a crumpled-up sweet-paper or playing patty-paws around the leg of a chair.

A soft toy has the additional advantage of always being there as company for the person with Alzheimer's.

> Growler probably made a greater difference to my mother's life than either my father or I did. He was never tired, never absented himself, and always said what my mother wanted to hear. The last is hardly surprising, since she herself was the source of his comments, always produced in a suitably growly voice to make clear that it was Growler who was speaking. Indeed, Growler became very much my mother's spokesperson. He would agree with whatever she said, help to reinforce her desires — for example, by stressing that he wanted to be taken with us on an outing and not left behind. He became the vehicle for expressing many of her thoughts. Growler's song, about liking a little bit of fuss made of him, is quoted at the end of this book.

> The following anecdote illustrates the complicity between my mother
> and Growler — in my father's words, they united in giving him stick:
>
> Bettie: *Why don't you sleep with me any more? You like sleeping with
> me, don't you Growler?'*
>
> Growler: *Yes, I do — very much!*

Avoiding treating the person like a child

An obvious objection to giving someone with Alzheimer's a soft toy or doll is
that we are treating them like a small child, and encouraging others to do the
same. This is indeed a risk, and one that we need to be careful to guard against.

> I had no problem about giving my mother Growler, because I knew
> that she had always had a special liking for old-fashioned teddy bears,
> and we had often played together with my bear, Edward, when I was
> grown up, long before the onset of her dementia.

Indeed, it is worth reminding yourself — and others — that a large number
of adults still keep their old toys and buy and display new ones too. Anne
Crawford, who was in charge of a large nursing home in Rotorua, New
Zealand, made a point of encouraging the members of her staff to give soft
toys as presents to one another for birthdays and Christmas to remind them
of this, and to prevent them looking down on residents who carried a
favourite toy about with them.

Against this possible disadvantage, too, one has to set the obvious benefits
that a toy provides in many cases. As Isabelle Vendeuvre, a speech therapist
in Paris, working predominantly with people who have dementia, said to
me recently, many of her patients who normally can't or won't speak will
actually comment on the puppet and other toys that she has in her office or
even begin a conversation with one of these.

> I often think of all the fun that my mother and I had with Growler,
> and the constant companionship and stimulus that he gave her. The
> final years of her life would have been much harder for her and us
> without him.

Making a suitable choice

Pets and toys are not for everyone but they are certainly worth considering. If you're getting a toy for someone, take their preferences into account. Anne Crawford had a range of different toy animals, so that residents could choose one that appealed or had some special relevance for them. Ideally the toy should be pleasant to touch, hard-wearing — and washable!

> Growler often got soup on his head, but my mother and I used to enjoy washing it off together. She would sit by the basin in her room with Growler on a towel on her lap while I gave him a going-over with a wet facecloth.

With a pet animal, its temperament is the major consideration. Other factors include the type of animal that the person is used to, and its size — not so small that you trip over it, but not so large that it costs a fortune to feed.

CHECKING AGAINST UNNECESSARY PROBLEMS

It is worth taking a moment before you begin any activity to ensure that factors unrelated to dementia aren't going to interfere with your time together.

- Are their glasses clean? Are they the right glasses?
- Is their hearing aid working?
- Do you need to find somewhere quiet to sit, without distractions, so that you can chat?

> One of my mother's favourite activities was going out in the garden. We got into the habit of checking her glasses, ensuring that she had been to the toilet recently and collecting her sunhat or a warm wrap, depending on the weather, so that we could stay out as long as she felt like it rather than having to come back inside too soon.

Physical discomfort may sometimes prevent the other person responding to our company. Something under their dentures or a sore throat may prevent them speaking; a full bladder, a stomach ache or bedsores may make them restless. A list of various physical problems is included in chapter 2 under the heading 'Factors that may be adding unnecessarily to the problem'.

FOCUS ON THE ESSENTIALS OF KEEPING IN TOUCH

You are both more likely to enjoy your time together if you keep the following points in mind:

- *Appreciate what you are doing together now rather than dwelling on the past or worrying about the future. Show the other person that you accept and like them as they are now.*

- *Remember that you are doing something worthwhile simply in being there for them. Your very presence communicates the fact that someone cares.*

- *Spending time with the person for whom you care, listening sympathetically to them, doing something together are all ways of making them feel valued. You are showing them that they are still someone worthy of attention and respect, despite their dementia.*

CHAPTER 4

THINGS TO DO TOGETHER

WHAT THIS CHAPTER COVERS

One of the questions that family carers frequently ask is, how on earth can I keep the person I care for amused? In this chapter I suggest some things that you can do together. The emphasis is on simple, everyday activities — none of them requires any special effort or expense. They are all ideas that worked with my mother or have worked for other carers.

THE OBJECT OF DOING THINGS TOGETHER

Pleasure

The highest priority in all the things you do together should be pleasure — doing something that you can both enjoy.

The point deserves stressing, to prevent us thinking of activities primarily in terms of their therapeutic value. Therapy has its place, but there are drawbacks to putting it first in our personal interactions with someone.

- The object of therapy is to maintain or improve various mental and bodily functions. **Orientation therapy**, for example, is designed to help people with dementia keep track of the here and now. It's fine for early stages of dementia. Later, it becomes too much a reminder of what the person has forgotten, what they cannot do. In all our interactions and throughout their dementia, maintaining their sense of wellbeing should be our major priority.

- Therapy is implicitly based on the assumption that the person for whom it is intended is deficient in some way. Although in a sense this is perfectly true of someone with Alzheimer's, it is difficult to maintain a positive relationship if we focus too much on what they can no longer do, or if we keep measuring them against their past capabilities. Instead, we need to enjoy simply being with them today.

Many of the activities that I suggest do have some obvious therapeutic benefits for the person with dementia, but enjoying yourselves is what counts. As the saying goes, laughter is the best medicine. And pleasure is the best therapy.

Participation

Another priority is participation. It is pleasant to feel that we belong — that we are part of what is happening around us. Unfortunately, though, people with dementia are all too often excluded. Former friends no longer visit; your family stop including you in activities; you get consigned to a separate, dementia wing of the nursing home so that you won't disturb the other residents or their visitors. This is indeed to be condemned to a form of living death. Hence the emphasis in the various activities that I suggest is on doing things together, and, as much as possible, making the person we care for feel that they are still a valued member of the living community.

Ideally, participation also involves playing an active role. Many amusements intended for the elderly or the dementing offer little more than something for them to watch or listen to. Yet the entertainment that my mother and her fellow residents probably enjoyed the most was not being sung to but singing together. And if we want to, we can usually find ways of including someone in an activity that is going on, even if their condition limits the type of participation that is possible for them. At the very least, we can show them that their presence adds something to the activity in question.

As mentioned in chapter 3, pets and soft toys can sometimes help a person with dementia to participate in what is going on around them.

As we will see in later chapters, active participation is important in making sense of what someone with Alzheimer's is saying and in understanding their stories. The underlying strategy recommended is sympathetic listening, which encourages the other person to take the star role of speaker and storyteller.

Making them feel valued

Every activity we undertake should make it clear that we value the other person. Showing them that we want to spend time with them is in itself valorising and there are many more specific ways in which we can make the other person feel that they have something to offer — that they are someone of importance in our eyes.

ENSURING THE OTHER PERSON'S PLEASURE

Since the overall object is to ensure the other person's pleasure, we need to keep some practical considerations in mind.

Consider their tastes and abilities

When choosing something to do together, it makes sense to keep both their tastes and abilities in mind.

> My mother had been an accomplished dressmaker, and still found it amusing to look through a fashion magazine with me. She enjoyed passing judgement on the various outfits (not to mention the models and their poses!), and I had plenty of ready-made opportunities to please her by commenting on the wonderful clothes that she had made for me.

Take no for an answer

Encourage them to do something that they enjoyed recently or that you think should amuse them, but don't overdo it. Learn to take no for an answer, as there will be days when they don't feel like participating or when we find it hard to come up with anything acceptable. Given that their condition has robbed them of most of their freedom and autonomy, it is important to consult their preferences as much as we possibly can.

Let them set the pace

Because of their condition, they will come to rely on us to suggest even simple activities, and to get them started, but we have to let them set the pace. Similarly, as soon as they get bored or tired, it is time to stop.

Try anything once

You never know what will work, until you try.

> I was surprised and delighted to find what a lasting success Growler was with my mother. Similarly, I wouldn't have thought of singing as an activity for her, since, as long as I could remember, she never sang,

> except in church and then in a rather reluctant and restrained manner.
> Yet singing became one of her greatest pleasures; some of the staff in the
> nursing home even thought that she must once have sung professionally.

Keep in mind that there may be pleasures just waiting to be discovered, or
rediscovered, and try anything once.

EVERYDAY PLEASURES

Everyday life provides a multitude of simple and inexpensive pleasures that
we can share with the person for whom we care.

The pleasure of simply doing nothing

Although this chapter is on things to do together, don't overlook the simple
pleasure of doing nothing! If the other person is daydreaming or resting, it
is enough to sit quietly with them. Often a sympathetic presence is all we
need to provide at such moments, reinforced perhaps by our holding or
gently stroking their hand.

Grooming

Pleasure, usefulness and relaxation are readily combined in routine acts
of grooming.

> My mother found it very soothing to have her hair brushed, and
> enjoyed feeling that she was being made look presentable.

Many daughters have told me that they assist their mothers by removing
unwanted facial whiskers — even in the advanced stages of dementia
enough personal vanity survives for this to be appreciated. Men with
dementia may have similar feelings about hairs growing on their ears. Hair
removal can be quite painful, though, as you probably realise, so you need
to talk reassuringly about what you are doing throughout the operation and
stop at once if the person starts to object. (One hair at a time, perhaps I
should add. I heard a horror story recently about a young nursing aide who,
without thinking, tried depilating a resident's upper lip with wax — the
screams and curses that this caused can be imagined.)

Giving a simple manicure and rubbing moisturising cream into the other person's hands is another simple grooming activity, and one that is easy to engage in even if you are unused to being demonstrative in public.

What you know of the past habits of the person for whom you care will suggest other forms of regular grooming that they will appreciate and that will help to preserve their sense of wellbeing and self-respect.

Don't overlook the pleasure that you can possibly give them by inviting them to reciprocate.

> I would ask my mother to do something straightforward such as giving my back a rub and she would be delighted to be able to do something for me.

Participating in everyday domestic tasks

Despite the fact that many daily household tasks gradually become too complicated for someone with Alzheimer's to carry out unaided, they may continue to enjoy being included in these activities.

First, though, it is worth taking a moment to consider whether any problems they are having with this sort of activity are partly caused by us. They may be perfectly capable of setting the table, for example, if we do the following:

- allow them the extra time that they require,

- provide prompts for each step so that they have only one task to worry about at a time, and

- don't get irked by the fact that they haven't arranged things as neatly as we would like.

Think how irritating it must be for someone who would like to help with these chores to be constantly told that we don't need their help — that they can't do this, or can't do it properly.

If their ability to participate is genuinely limited, there are still ways of including them and making them feel useful.

My mother enjoyed having her routine offers to assist me accepted, even if she did no more than carry the napkins to the table. Similarly, she regularly handed me the clothes pegs when I was hanging out the washing. Noting the colours of the pegs and counting them provided her with additional amusement while doing this.

Sometimes it is important to have equipment that is familiar to them and hence easy to use.

The staff of a specialised dementia wing in a hospital in Nantes in France refused to give up their old brooms and mops because they knew that the residents felt comfortable using these. The smart new cleaning machine favoured by the health authorities might do the job better, and more hygienically but it would rob those residents who liked to help with the housework of their chance to feel useful and at home. The sensible solution, which kept everyone happy, proved to be allowing the residents to sweep and mop in the morning, and having the new machine go over the areas separately later in the day.

Even when the ability to participate actively is considerably reduced, we can still help people to feel included in what is going on.

When my mother was still living at home and I was preparing a meal I would discuss with her what I was doing, and ask for her advice and comments — thereby acknowledging her past skills in cooking. I would also bring things to show her — 'Look how fresh these peas are, you can still see the moisture on them. Here, taste one!' We might shell the peas together, and even if my mother managed to shell only one or two pods or she ate more peas than she shelled or she simply turned a pod over and over in her hands, what did this matter to me compared with her obvious pleasure in joining in? An activity like cooking also provided an opportunity for me to reminisce about meals she had cooked for us in the past and so reinforce her sense of personal identity and past achievements.

Even when active participation is virtually impossible, being where things are happening can help give a person the sense of being in contact with daily life. Professional carers in specialised homes have noted that the most popular sitting places for residents are usually those where they can see what is going on — by the entrance, for example.

The sights, smells and sounds of various activities also act as a stimulus and may well prompt old memories to resurface.

> I recall a discussion about this at an Alzheimer's Association conference, in which one professional carer shared with us what happened when the ironing room was being repainted and the ironing had to be temporarily moved to the main lounge. The once familiar sight of someone ironing, the distinctive odour of freshly ironed cotton, and the creak of the ironing board and hiss of the steam got residents sharing reminiscences about the past, all triggered by this simple activity happening in their midst.

We tend to overlook the extent to which being frail or having dementia tends to exclude people from a whole range of normal, everyday physical sensations — so much so, that they could be seen as suffering from sensory deprivation. This helps to explain the success of 'memory workshops' (or 'reminiscence sessions') in which people are given the opportunity to look at, touch, hear, smell or taste a range of once familiar items.

> Loic Laine, who used to run such workshops in Angers, France, told me how the smell of wattle inspired one elderly nursing home resident to talk about his former experiences as a carpenter working with acacia wood; another was reminded of his old primary school teacher by the smell of lavender.

This suggests the value of enhancing various experiences for the person we care for by bringing a range of senses into play — as I was doing when I invited my mother to look at, touch and taste the fresh peas, for example. Moreover, such reinforcement may well help messages to get through to someone affected by dementia.

The 'cuppa' and other rituals

The normal round of daily activities tends to be punctuated by a number of ritual pauses. We take time out from housework or gardening or from our job to have a cup of morning tea, for example. Another ritual in our household was the glass of wine or fruit juice and something to nibble before the evening meal. These are simple pleasures that everyone can enjoy together.

> I much appreciated the fact that the home where my mother lived for the final years of her life set store by the rituals of morning and afternoon tea and included any visitors as a matter of course.

Other daily rituals include such things as listening to the news or watching some favourite TV program, or taking the dog for a walk before bedtime. Such routine moments have additional benefits for people with dementia. The routines help to orient them towards the cycle of the day and its pattern of activities. Certain rituals, like the little something before dinner, help to stimulate their appetite and prepare them for the meal to come. Similarly, the routines associated with getting ready for bed prepare them for going to sleep.

Everyday amusements

As well as these routine moments of time off, there are many entertainments that we engage in most days and which may well become part of our daily ritual.

- Feeding the birds is both routine and entertaining for some people.

> My mother and the other residents in the home regularly put out the breakfast crumbs for the sparrows, both for the fun of watching their antics and also for the satisfaction of offering something and having it so willingly accepted.

- Pets or toys are a valuable source of amusement and activity for many people with dementia and their carers too. Pets can be fed, groomed or stroked, and taken for walks; they provide company and a readily available topic for conversation. Toys offer most of these, and have the added advantage of always being available and never getting tired.

- Going for a walk together is another simple activity. There is always something to notice and talk about and the fresh air and exercise are good for both of you.

> My mother particularly appreciated spending time out in the grounds around the nursing home. Because there were plenty of pleasant spots to sit and winding paths suitable for wheelchairs, we were able to enjoy the garden with her even when her mobility had become severely limited.

- If the weather is not suitable for going outside, try looking through a book or magazine together.

> A coffee table book with pictures to comment on, or a fashion magazine, were usually successful in capturing my mother's interest. I would be guided in my choices by whatever had some relevance to her past life and so would provide me with opportunities to remind her of things that she had achieved. The clothes we admired in a fashion magazine, for example, gave me the chance to boast on her behalf about the lovely dresses that she had made me. A favourite story, which she never tired of hearing, was of how I had worn one of her dresses to a special party and had been asked if it had come from Paris. 'No,' I replied, *'my mother made it for me.'*

- Most families have stock stories which get trotted out regularly whenever there is a family get-together.

> My father discovered that the old stories about some of my childhood misdeeds were almost always a success with my mother. Such stories tend to become ritualised and are reassuringly familiar. My mother would clearly be waiting for the punch-line, and enjoy it when it came. These particular stories also helped to reaffirm the relationship between my parents and to remind my mother of my existence when I was absent.

- Old photographs are another source of interest, and can trigger memories of the past. A number of books for carers recommend helping someone in the earlier stages of Alzheimer's to put together a scrapbook covering their life. This provides a comforting reminder of what they have achieved at a time when their identity is beginning to be threatened;

later it becomes a valuable talking point with family and friends and a means of filling in other carers on their background. Putting together an account of one's life is an interesting and valorising activity for older people who don't have dementia too. Writing his memoirs gave my father something positive and absorbing to focus his thoughts on during the long period of my mother's decline.

> My mother also had stories to tell me about her past although, as her dementia advanced, the stories became increasingly fantastic mixtures of past and present, real and unreal people and events. Nevertheless, listening to these stories can be a rewarding experience — not least for the pleasure that being listened to gives the person telling the story. I particularly like the suggestion that we should regard such reminiscences, irrespective of whether they are true or not, 'as a form of personalised gift'. [xi]

- A 'rainy day special' can be going through drawers or a wardrobe.

> With my mother, this was more fun than it sounds. Each occasion was something of a discovery for her. She would forget what she actually had and sometimes be anxious that she had no clothes other than what she was wearing, so the contents of drawers and wardrobe came as a pleasant surprise. Many of the garments were ones that she had made; she also had quite a collection of shawls and scarves that I and other friends had given her. Hence I had plenty of opportunities for recalling pleasant memories and giving my mother's ego a boost. Another, practical benefit was that I was able to review the state of her clothing.

- Singing, reciting familiar poems or nursery rhymes, and dancing are routine, rhythmic activities, and hence able to be enjoyed by people with dementia even if their mobility and speech is extremely limited. Such activities are usually part of the regular program in nursing homes and day care centres, but can obviously be engaged in at home too. They are also activities that someone with Alzheimer's can share with young members of their family. Dancing is a good way of getting exercise on days when it is too wet and cold to go outside. Most music shops have tapes and CDs of old-time dance music.

One woman whom I met at an Alzheimer's Association conference told me that the easiest way to encourage her husband to move from one part of the house to the other was to invite him to dance with her. At times when he refused to walk into the dining room, for instance, he would happily waltz there.

Some form of participation in such activities is possible even when someone is in a very advanced stage of dementia. I have seen people who spend much of the day chair-bound and shrunk in on themselves brighten up and move their bodies in time to the music during sing-along sessions.

Old nursery rhymes, such as 'Sing a song of sixpence' and 'Baa baa black sheep', became a key source of interaction with my mother during the final months of her life. Even when she was on her deathbed, she would still murmur a response when my father chanted the opening line to her.

- Simple ball games and various types of children's game may also provide amusement for some people. Do such things together in a light-hearted way, as families often do when they are on a picnic; this helps to prevent the activity from infantilising the person with dementia. Sometimes watching you and other family members trying to keep a balloon in the air, for example, may stimulate them to join in.

- Chatting together is part of most of these activities, and is often activity enough in itself. Even if someone with dementia shows little sign of responding, continue to speak to them and to include them in conversations. Always assume that they are listening and able to understand you, because this may well be true.

Everyday outings

There were various outings that my mother continued to enjoy. My father regularly drove her to a pleasant lakeside park where they could feed the seagulls. He also often took her and her friend Wally out to morning or afternoon tea. He chose a quiet time during the week and day for this, and the visits always passed without incident. Sometimes he would drive to a scenic spot where there was an ice cream van and buy them all ice creams. As well, we were particularly fortunate in having a number of friends who cared sufficiently for my mother to continue to invite us around for morning or afternoon tea.

Many outings that are part of everyday life remain possible for longer than one might expect, especially if you choose an appropriate time and place for them.

My mother and I sometimes indulged in window shopping at a quiet time of day or when the shops were shut. We also went shopping together. Mrs David, from whom my parents had always bought their fruit and vegetables, continued to greet my mother warmly and make her feel welcome. Sometimes we went shopping for clothes. I would choose a smaller, more specialised shop. This was potentially less confusing, since it stocked only the sort of item that we were after (underwear, for instance), and it was much easier to get my mother into and out of. When mobility became a problem, our friends Neil and Olwen would sometimes drive my mother into town and park in front of an interesting shop. My mother would enjoy chatting with them about the passers by, and if she became bored or agitated it was easy to move on.

Many French nursing homes for people with dementia regularly organise normal outings for their residents, taking them to restaurants, shops, markets and even the cinema. How to behave on such occasions is deeply ingrained in our long-term memory for procedures that we have performed many times before, which is why even people with advanced dementia can surprise us by conducting themselves appropriately. Moreover, continuing to give them the opportunity to engage in such activities helps to keep these semi-automatic social skills alive. An important factor in the success of these outings though is our own attitude. Given the sensitivity of people with dementia to our body language, they may well pick up on and react to our feelings of nervousness, anxiety or embarrassment about being in public with them.

TREATS, SPECIAL OCCASIONS AND CELEBRATIONS

As well as the everyday pleasures and activities suggested above, there are treats, special occasions and family or national celebrations in which someone with Alzheimer's can participate.

Treats

By treats, I mean enjoyable events that don't happen every day. Examples are my mother's invitations to morning and afternoon tea at a friend's house; the picnics on which other close friends used to take her; and my visits, which usually lasted for at least a week. Another example is the weekly outing to have 'a cup of real coffee, like they make in Vienna' which a migrant family arranged for their mother who was in care. The regular visit to an Austrian-style cafe was keenly appreciated, and provided a crucial reinforcement of her identity for this woman.

Often part of the pleasure of such treats is looking forward to them and then talking about them afterwards. Despite their memory problems, someone with Alzheimer's can engage in this aspect too, with a little tactful help from us. Indeed, if the treat is sufficiently central to the person's sense of identity, as the cafe visit was, the person may need little or no prompting to recall and talk about it. However, we need to be cautious here, as such conversations may be distressful rather than pleasant for someone who is still painfully aware of their tendency to forget things.

Special occasions and festivals

The year is also marked by a number of special occasions and festivals — birthdays and other anniversaries, Christmas, key national holidays, key events in the religious calendars of particular faiths. These are highly ritualised activities, ones that may well be much easier for someone with Alzheimer's to participate in than one-off, unusual events. Regular, well-known festivities usually offer plenty of opportunity to include someone, however severely they may be handicapped. Depending upon their own wishes and abilities, that person can take part in the preparations, for example. They can help in some way with cooking for Christmas and setting up the table and decorating the tree. At the very least, they can be encouraged to share with us their memories of Christmas from when they were a child, or asked for their advice about the placement of a decoration. There are various ways of including them in the conversation and showing them that their presence is adding to our pleasure in the occasion.

Time as a cycle of seasonal events

These key events of the year have the added advantage of helping someone with Alzheimer's stay oriented towards the cycle of the seasons. Even though they may have lost their sense of time as a linear sequence, from their earliest memories to the present day, and can no longer tell you what year it is, the repeated cycle of seasonal events is still potentially meaningful for them, precisely because of its repeated and ritualised nature. Each season, and each seasonal event has its own particular signs — things we can notice, touch, taste and talk about together.

CHAPTER 5

MAKING SENSE OF WHAT THEY SAY

WHAT THIS CHAPTER COVERS

Interacting with someone who has Alzheimer's disease becomes more difficult once their speech starts being affected by their condition. In this chapter I concentrate on the typical changes in their speech and on strategies for continuing to understand what they are saying, despite these changes.

- *The first section stresses the importance of being a good listener. By listening, we are showing the other person that we still value them. Moreover, however little we manage to grasp of what they are saying, we should at least be able to recognise the feelings 'behind the words'.*

- *The second section suggests how to identify what the other person is actually talking about.*

- *Recognising their topic and its relevance for them helps us to respond appropriately, as the three examples of conversations given in the third section demonstrate.*

- *The fourth section covers strategies for making sense of the words that people with Alzheimer's use. Even though their use of language changes, it does so in a systematic way. If we know the rules of their new language, it becomes easier for us to work out the meaning of what they are saying. A key strategy here is to realise that their words are usually linked in some way with the words that would normally be used, and to recognise the significance of these links.*

- *The final section gives another example to demonstrate that the words of someone with Alzheimer's are rarely meaningless, if we make the attempt to understand what they are trying to say.*

THE VALUE OF LISTENING

Show them that they are worth listening to

By listening, you are showing the other person that they are still worth listening to. Indeed, your very act of listening helps to prevent the 'loss of self' which is often associated with dementia. People with Alzheimer's are in danger of losing their social identity, because that very identity depends on other people responding positively to them. Simply by listening to someone with Alzheimer's, then, you are acknowledging them as a person and confirming their social identity as a speaker who gets listened to. By not bothering to listen, on the other hand, you imply that they have no value — they are nobody.

Being a good listener

Show the other person that you are indeed listening to them and that you are interested in whatever they are trying to tell you. You can show this just as you do with someone who doesn't have dementia, although you may need to be more obvious about it to make sure that your attention registers with them.

- Demonstrate your interest by being close to the other person, perhaps holding their hand, and by looking at their face.

- Ums, nods, exclamations and hand squeezes will show that you are paying attention.

- Repeating a key word or phrase, and asking questions about what they are saying will also show that you are trying to understand them. (The section on recognising what they are talking about will help you to come up with appropriate questions here.)

Identify and respond to the feeling behind the words

By listening to someone in this way, at the very least you should be able to identify the feeling behind their words. Certain repeated phrases, the tone of their voice, their general body language will indicate the emotional content of what they are saying, even if you can't identify exactly what the emotion is about.

Identifying the feeling behind the words is a crucial strategy in all our dealings with other people.

> When my father, who is far from dementing, telephones me, I pay attention to his tone of voice, knowing that this will tell me more about the way he feels than what he actually says to me.

Realising whether the other person is feeling happy — or sad, or agitated — tells you how to respond to what they are saying. Like anyone else, someone with Alzheimer's wants us to sympathise with their feelings

> My mother was right to be cross with me for singing 'Oh what a beautiful morning' when she was in a bad mood.

RECOGNISING WHAT THEY ARE TALKING ABOUT

Identifying the feeling behind the words gives you your first important clue as to what someone with Alzheimer's is talking about. You know whether it is a subject that makes them feel happy, sad, or agitated. This emotion is itself an essential part of what they are trying to tell you. Once you have grasped the underlying emotion, ask yourself what might be causing it.

The immediate context may provide a clue

Sometimes the immediate context will give you the necessary clue.

- If the person is in a strange and potentially threatening place, such as a doctor's surgery or a room full of unfamiliar medical equipment, their agitation may well be caused by their surroundings. Indeed, because of their memory problems, even a setting that we might expect to be familiar to them may seem strange and threatening.

- The context may be reminding them of something from the past. If they are looking at a Christmas tree and crying, for example, it may well be because they are missing the family Christmases of their childhood, or even because something bad once happened to them at this time of year.

Their past history may provide clues too

Often the secret to understanding what someone with Alzheimer's is saying or doing lies in knowing their past history.

This was true of the man mentioned in chapter 1, who was following the bed-makers and throwing the freshly arranged bedcovers up in the air. The clue to this bizarre behaviour was that he had worked as a wool-classer and was repeating the routine gestures of throwing a sheep's fleece onto a table.

The past also provides the clue to explaining why one woman believed that there were no children around 'because they have all been killed'. When I tell you that she was living in a nursing home run by the Jewish community in Melbourne and that many of the residents were Holocaust survivors, you will immediately understand what she was talking about. My Melbourne colleagues, who told me about her[xii] encouraged staff and family members to bring their children to visit the home so that this woman and the other residents could see that there were indeed still children in the world.

Another example, which I will be giving in full at the end of this section, is that of a woman who was wandering around crying and asking people if they had seen her mother. Long-dead people and past events are often part of the present reality of people with Alzheimer's.

Knowing about a person's past may also provide valuable clues for understanding the stories that they tell us.

Finding the relevant frame of reference

What we have been doing in the above examples is identifying the other person's frame of reference. We need to ask ourselves, what event or topic are they referring to? And to what time and place?

Normally the answers to these questions are clear. For example, we say *'This hospital gives me the creeps'* or *'That reminds me of something that happened to me in my childhood'* and in so doing tell our listeners that we are referring to this hospital, now and the creepy feelings that it is giving us, or to some event in our past. Similarly, an introductory comment such as *'Wouldn't it be nice if we won a million dollars'* lets people know that we are imagining something — not reporting on a real event. However, someone who has

Alzheimer's often doesn't give us these clues; instead, we may have to work out for ourselves what their frame of reference is at the moment.

Unfortunately, not everyone bothers to find out what someone with Alzheimer's is talking about. In a study of conversations between normal people and someone with dementia Hollis Bohling discovered that most people either stick with their own frame of reference or simply give up on the conversation altogether.[xiii] However, if we want the conversation to continue and to be of interest to the other person, we need to be more sensitive to their frame of reference. We can use simple questions to help establish the when and where that they are talking about and to test whether we have grasped the essentials of the topic that interests them. One of the examples below demonstrates this.

Respecting their frame of reference

Once we have recognised what someone with Alzheimer's is talking about, we should respect that frame of reference. We need to show them that we understand and sympathise with their feelings and memories. This applies even when the feelings and memories are sad ones. Note how the carer in the first example below validates Bridget's feelings of missing her mother before attempting to soothe her or re-involve her in the group activities.

Similarly, if the other person has found a subject that interests them it makes sense to encourage them to keep talking about this rather than changing the topic or introducing elements that are irrelevant to them. After all, we all prefer to be talking about something that matters to us, as my mother makes clear in the final example below.

EXAMPLES

The following examples of conversations with someone who has dementia show carers using the strategies that I have just been discussing.

Responding to the woman who was crying for her mother

My first example comes from a book for professional carers by Tom Kitwood. It shows how a professional caregiver at a day care centre responded to a woman who was walking about crying and asking if anyone had seen her mother. The carer joins 'Bridget' and starts talking to her:

'Are you looking for your mother?'

'Yes, have you seen her? I want to go home. I want my mother.'

'What does she look like?'

'She looks . . . ummm . . . normal looking.'

'Was she a big woman or small?'

'She's normal. Where is she? I want my mother.'

'Do you miss her?'

'Yes,' Bridget cried. *'Take me home. I want my mother. Where's my mother?'*

'I'm sorry Bridget,' the careworker said softly, *'she's not here.'*

Bridget cried as the careworker gave Bridget a hug.

'If your mother was here what would she do?' *'Nice things.'*

'Would she give you a nice cuddle? Would you like me to give you a nice cuddle?'

'Yes.'

They cuddled and the careworker led Bridget over to a sofa where they sat. The careworker held Bridget and smoothed down her hair.

'I'm sure your mother loved you very much, and you were a very good daughter to her.'

'Yes, and I love her very much. And I love you.'

'Well, I'm right here with you, Bridget.'[xiv]

Soon after this Bridget was ready to join in the group activities in the day care centre.

In this example the person with Alzheimer's can still speak normally but the caregiver needs to work out why she is crying for her mother. We can guess that Bridget's behaviour relates both to her present context and her past history — she is feeling lost and anxious just as she may have done on her first day at a new school or play centre.

Note how the caregiver responds to the situation:

- She immediately acknowledges Bridget's frame of reference by asking if she is looking for her mother. Her questions show Bridget that her search for her mother is being taken seriously; her frame of reference is being treated with respect.

- The carer then checks that she has correctly identified the emotion underlying Bridget's search — she misses her mother.

- At this point (rather than at the start of their exchange) the carer gently breaks the news that the mother isn't there, softening the impact with a hug.

- Her next questions show that she is trying to find out how her mother's presence would have helped Bridget. As she had suspected, Bridget needs some motherly affection, which she is able to give her.

Contrast this exchange with what might have happened if the carer had ignored Bridget's feelings and immediately told her that her mother was unavailable, or dead. Bridget would almost certainly have become even more unhappy and agitated.

Finding a common topic of conversation

The next example comes from Hollis Bohling's study of conversations with people who have Alzheimer's. In this case the person has difficulty speaking normally. The carer makes an effort to start up a conversation by introducing a specific topic — Chicago in winter.

Caregiver: *'Chicago's cold!'*

Patient: *'Oh, yeah.'*

Caregiver: *'The winter's cooool. You drive your car and slide around on the snow and ice.'*

Patient: *'Yeah, what bothers me (I go to try it, and do it) is my wife...'*

Caregiver: *'Um-hum.'*

Patient: *'Is a . . . is a . . . Won't be able to go up that hill.'*

Caregiver: *'Won't be able to go up the hill?'*

> Patient: 'The hill ... I mean, I wouldn't make too much of it. Change to ... cause, I — I ... twisted, twisted. You gotta get up, clean that walk, so you can get out and get ... and then from there, just let it.'
>
> Caregiver: 'Yeah.'
>
> Patient: 'I'm not kidding.'
>
> Caregiver: 'Imagine it's hard to drive up the hill when it snows, huh?'
>
> Patient: 'Yeah.'
>
> Caregiver: 'Boy, yeah.'
>
> Patient: 'That's what, that's what.' [xv]

- The patient's 'what bothers me' shows that he is introducing a personal frame of reference.

- The carer's responses ('um-hum', repeating the patient's words in a questioning tone of voice, and 'yeah') show that he is listening and trying to grasp what the other person is talking about. (Bohling notes that the carer can't be sure whether the patient is talking about winter in Chicago or something else, which could be in the past. However, his responses encourage the patient to continue talking.)

- When the carer thinks he has identified what the patient is now talking about, he checks that he has got it right.

- Finally both carer and patient recognise that they are talking about the same topic and emphasise their agreement about it.

Another carer, and especially one with some knowledge of the patient's recent history, might have picked up on the earlier clue provided by the reference to his wife. As Bohling suggests,

> the thought of driving a car may have triggered the memory that his wife will not let him drive any more.

However, what is most important in this example is that the person with Alzheimer's has been encouraged to continue speaking by his listener's response. As a result, the conversation does get somewhere.

Contrast what would have happened if the carer had continued to talk about winter in Chicago and made no effort to involve the patient or to understand his contributions to the conversation.

Encouraging my mother's singing story

My third example comes from a recorded conversation between me and my mother. She is telling me about a recent singing exploit. (Incidentally, this story is substantially true — just worked up a bit to make it worth telling me.) I had heard this story several times already, but respond as if I am hearing it for the first time. This makes telling me more fun for my mother and encourages her to continue. (Of course, having already heard the story actually helps me to make appropriate comments!) My mother (Bettie) had just started her story again when I switched on the tape recorder.

> Jane: *'No, I wasn't here last night — what happened?'*
>
> Bettie: *'There was a collection of people who came and sang.'*
>
> Jane: *'What did they sing?'*
>
> Bettie: *'Several songs . . . and I couldn't resist . . . '*
>
> Jane: *'What did you do?'*
>
> Bettie: *'I sang as loudly as I could!'*
>
> Jane: *'Oh dear! Did you drown them out?'*
>
> Bettie: *'Yes, very nearly. And then they came and said how much they'd enjoyed my beautiful singing!'*
>
> Jane: *'Oh, gosh!'* (We both laugh.)

- Note that I respond to the implied invitation to be impressed by this story (*'Oh, dear! Gosh!'*).

- My question, *'Did you drown them out?'*, picks up on a detail of the story that my mother had already told me about with obvious relish.

At this point a visitor joins us. Note that at first the visitor introduces another aspect of the same event, but it is one that doesn't really interest my mother, because her singing story is about <u>her</u>.

Bettie (to visitor): *'Did you hear me singing last night?'*

Visitor: *'Jennifer Jones was here singing last night.'*

Bettie: *'Who?'*

Visitor: *'Jennifer Jones was here singing.'*

Bettie: *'What was she singing for?'*

Visitor: *'Well, I don't think she was singing for her supper. She was with a group of people and they came and sang to you last night.'*

Bettie: *'It was a group of people ... I must be thinking of something different. It was a selected group of people and they'd come here singing.'*

Visitor: *'I see. Did you sing too?'*

Bettie: *'I sang as loudly as I could.'* (We all three laugh.)

Visitor: *'Jolly good!'*

- If I played you the tape of this conversation you could tell from my mother's tone of voice exactly what she meant by her response to the introduction of a new character into her story. Her *'Who?'* implies *'who the hell is this person'* and her *'what . . .' 'what the hell is she doing in my singing story!'*

- She then decides that she and the visitor are talking about *'different'* singing episodes.

- The visitor by now realises that his comments aren't helping the conversation and so he encourages her to continue with her own story — which she does for most of the rest of that side of the tape.

A REMINDER: In all these examples the person with Alzheimer's is still capable of speaking, even if in one case this is only in fragments. Don't forget the point made at the start of this chapter — *even if we can't understand anything of what the person is saying, our act of listening shows them that they are still someone who deserves to be listened to.*

MAKING SENSE OF THEIR WORDS

Most of the strategies just discussed are obviously much easier to apply if the person for whom we care is still using words more or less normally. However, one of the effects of Alzheimer's disease is that this becomes increasingly difficult, as in the case in the middle example above. In the section that follows I will outline strategies for making sense of someone whose speech has already become affected by their condition. As you will see, apparently ill-chosen or meaningless words and fragments of speech still have a core of meaning to them, which we can work out if we know the rules that their language now follows.

The links between 'wrong' and right words

Someone with Alzheimer's often has trouble finding the right word. We have already seen an example of this in the 'wrong' responses to the sketch of a beaver. However, this example also showed that there were obvious links between the wrong answers (rat, fish) and the right word (beaver). Beavers live in the water, like fish; and they look rather like large rats — the one in the sketch certainly did.

Detailed studies have been done of the naming errors made by people with dementia. These studies demonstrate that links between the word used and the correct word are very common; in fact they are usually readily identifiable in at least two errors out of three. [xvi]

To illustrate the links between apparently wrong answers and the correct word, I have listed below some of the ways in which my mother referred to bananas. These were one of her favourite fruits, and my father often brought her one when he made his daily visit. It became quite a game between them for him to ask, '*What's this?*' and for her to come up with a reply. Normally it is not a good idea to ask someone with Alzheimer's a question that they will have trouble answering, but my mother clearly enjoyed the ritual and sometimes responded playfully. '*You tell me, and then I'll tell you,*' she said with a chuckle on one occasion; on another, when my father seemed surprised by the answer she'd given, she added, '*You were expecting me to say something ridiculous, so I did!*'

Here are some of my mother's names for a banana:

1. 'a nice thing you put in your mouth'

2. 'a persimmon'

3. 'a yellow cucumber'

4. 'Mrs David'

All these alternative names are linked to bananas, even the last one!

Most of the links here are fairly obvious:

1. In the first answer the fruit is linked with what you do with it (put it in your mouth); it belongs to the general category of things that we eat, and, more specifically, things that my mother liked to eat.

2. In the second, it is linked with another type of fruit and, again, a fruit that my mother also liked very much.

3. In the third, it is linked with a broader general category, fruit and vegetables. Even more obvious, though, is a link of likeness — some cucumbers are banana shaped, and a yellow one would indeed look like a banana.

4. The fourth answer refers to the fact that for years we purchased most of our fruit and vegetables from Mrs David. The association was reinforced by our habit of commenting on *'the excellent bananas (strawberries, radishes, lettuce etc) that we get from Mrs David.'* This example demonstrates that links may exist in those cases where they aren't at all obvious.

I'll now cover each type of link in more detail, specifying the questions that you can ask to help you identify the link and thus work out the meaning underlying what the person has said.

Assume that there is a link

The first strategy is obvious. Assume that there is some link between what the person is saying and what they are trying to tell us, and look for that link! As my mother's names for banana have just shown, even bizarre choices are usually linked in some way with the word that they should have used.

- *Ask yourself, what links this word with the one they should be using?*

Look for links of likeness

A yellow cucumber looks like a banana. There is an obvious similarity between the item my mother has named and the banana to which she is actually referring. Such links are very common and usually fairly easy to recognise.

Another example reminds us to look for links of likeness even when these are not so obvious.

> On one occasion my mother called the hospital cat a *'seagull'*. Seeing my father's surprised reaction, she added, *'Of course it's a seagull — it's black and white.'* Indeed it was, just like the black-backed gulls that she enjoyed feeding during regular outings to the lakeside park.

Often these links of likeness are expressed by giving the one name to a range of similar items.

> One woman whose naming errors have been studied was using the word 'dog' to refer not only to dogs but to other small, hairy, four-legged animals as well. [xvii] For her, 'dog' now meant 'dog-like'. Small children do much the same thing, using a word they know — 'horse', for example — whenever they see a cow or a sheep. My mother tended to call any small, furry animal that she liked a 'bear'. Cats, small dogs, lambs were all like her beloved Growler.

In these examples, the person's mind is working in terms of general categories — horse-like, dog-like, bear-like things. I'll be discussing the relevance of such general categories further in a moment.

> • *Ask yourself, is there a link of likeness? Does the word make better sense if I add 'like this in some way'?*

Links of likeness may express an attitude or emotion

> When my mother called other animals 'bears' she was also expressing her feelings about them. *'Look at the dear little bear,'* she would say, pointing at the small dog accompanying a visitor. The name was

> wrong but her meaning was clear — she was pleased to see an animal
> that was small and cuddly, like her teddy bear. Rather than telling her
> that it wasn't a bear, we would reply, *'Yes, isn't it a dear little animal'*
> or *'Yes, isn't it a dear little dog.'*

Recognising the feelings underlying misnamings is an excellent way of
coping with being called by the wrong name yourself.

> Sometimes my mother called my father 'Howard' instead of his real
> name, 'Tom'. This didn't upset him, because he was aware of the links
> of likeness between himself and Howard and the feelings that went
> with them. Howard was my mother's dearly loved older brother, who
> had died a few years previously. My mother may have forgotten my
> father's name but she still recognised him as someone who was
> important to her.

> Something very similar was happening when the father of a friend of
> mine started calling his daughter 'mother'. His daughter did indeed
> resemble her grandmother when a young woman, as family photos
> showed; and her father probably remembered his mother as she was
> then rather than as the white-haired old lady that she eventually became.
> Even without the physical similarity, though, there was an emotional
> one. The daughter was loving and caring, just as his mother had been.
> The misnaming was a recognition of this likeness, and a response to the
> daughter's motherly attentions. Rather than thinking, *'He no longer
> knows who I am'* the daughter could take comfort in still being
> recognised by her father as a caring member of his immediate family.

- *Look for any links of likeness, and ask yourself, what feelings
  do these links of likeness express?*

A note about responding to use of the wrong word

Carers often ask me how they should respond to a person's use of the wrong
word for something. In particular they want to know whether they should

correct the errors, and, conversely, whether they should start using the wrong word themselves.

If the person is in a sufficiently early stage of the dementing process, they may welcome being corrected. Later, though, it can be counterproductive to insist on drawing attention to the errors they are making. Indeed, this may well suggest that you are more interested in finding fault than in listening to what they have to say.

> I never corrected my mother's naming errors openly. I did find, though, that if I used the correct name in my reply to her — for instance, *'dear little dog'*, rather than *'dear little bear'* — she would sometimes follow suit and start calling it a dog too.

I would recommend this as a more tactful way of reminding the person of the word that would normally be used.

Neither my father nor I ever used my mother's new words for things in talking to her. There didn't seem to be any need for this, since she was still able to recognise and understand the normal name. Words that belong to their youth or to the private vocabulary that families sometimes develop are another matter, however. These are discussed below under 'Recognising words from the past'.

> • *Respond to the meaning that the word has for them, rather than to the word itself.*

Thinking in broader categories

In many of the examples just given, the person is thinking in terms of a broad category — things they like to eat, dog-like animals, people that are important in their lives. Again, there is plenty of evidence that this is how the thought processes of people with Alzheimer's work. The general categories still exist in their minds, but items within each category become interchangeable.

In chapter 2 I compared this to what happens when we reach into a familiar cupboard in the dark. Instead of the item that we are reaching for we may well grab one stored nearby. Thus, when my mother needed a name for banana, she came up with that of another of her favourite fruits, or with what you actually do with such things — put them in your mouth. When she needed a name for one of her favourite animals, 'bear' tended to pop into her mind first.

> • **Ask yourself, what general category of person, event or thing are they talking about?**

Combining several items into one

Another thing that often happens to items that belong to the same category is that they become combined.

> When my mother told me a story about Willy, her pet sheep, her memories of him had become mixed in with memories of other pets, including fictional ones such as Mr Ed the talking horse. Willy was now a superpet — one pet made up of all these memories. Similarly, memories of the different gardens that she had developed were stored together in her mind and would come to the surface when we were enjoying a walk in the hospital grounds. She would tell us about how she had arranged the rocks in the rockery that we had just admired. This garden and all those others she had known in the past had become one and the same as far as she was concerned.

Recognising these combinations as such and accepting the mixture of fact and fantasy that sometimes goes into them are valuable strategies for making sense of the stories people like my mother tell us too.

> • **Have several items in the general category become combined into one?**

Links between words that occur together

Another very common type of link is that which exists between words that usually get spoken together.

> One example of this is my mother calling the banana 'Mrs David'. Whenever we spoke about fruit and vegetables we tended to mention Mrs David's name too. Hence Mrs David and the names of fruit had become closely linked in our minds.
>
> The example I like best of links between words is my mother's greeting to her favourite nurse — *'Hello Redbreast!'* Most people with whom I have shared this immediately guess the nurse's correct name — Robyn. Robin Redbreast is such a common combination of words that one of them immediately reminds us of the other. The link was reinforced in this case by a link of likeness too. Robyn Thomas, the nurse in question, was wearing her usual red cardigan — so both the robins were red. Robyn was clearly delighted with the very appropriate substitute name that my mother had found for her.

The close association that develops between words that are repeatedly said or sung together helps people with Alzheimer's to sing and recite well-known pieces. Once they hear the tune or the opening words, they have little trouble in coming up with what follows. These familiar pieces have been repeated so often that they have become firmly lodged in procedural memory, the type of memory that best resists the effects of dementia.

We can draw on the links between words that usually go together to help make sense of the fragments spoken by people with advanced dementia. As the example at the end of this chapter demonstrates, we can complete these fragments by filling in whatever would normally go together with them. What could be the meaning of *'A first day for a child . . .'*? *'First day at school'* is a familiar enough expression and one that makes sense in this particular context.

> • *Ask yourself, what word or words are usually said with this one?*
>
> • *Can I use them to complete this fragment?*

Recognising words from the past

Often what someone with Alzheimer's is saying or doing makes sense if we relate it to their past. This also applies to words that they may be using.

Just as past memories rise to the surface and become part of the present, so do words from the past. An obvious example of this is the way people for whom English is a second language eventually revert to their mother tongue.

> The residents of the Jewish nursing home in Melbourne come from a number of different European countries and many now speak in their original language, especially when they are excited or agitated about something. One of the residents has a particularly impressive stock of Russian swearwords![xviii]

Even if someone has always spoken English, some of the words that they use may have been current when they were young or may belong to the private vocabulary that sometimes develops within a family.

> My mother had the vocabulary of an educated Englishwoman brought up in the early decades of the twentieth century, and traces of this remained even when she was dementing. The assistant who typed up the tapes I had made of our conversations was Australian and belonged to a different generation; hence she had to guess at some of the words that my mother occasionally used. The fact that she sometimes guessed wrongly brought home to me the relevance of taking someone's age and background into account when trying to understand what they are saying.

My mother's pet name for me — her 'ewe lamb' — is an example of the private vocabulary that families sometimes develop. The usefulness of knowing these special expressions is demonstrated by an incident that Mitra Khosravi includes in her book for French-speaking carers. [xix]

> A woman that Mitra was helping care for had become incontinent. She made no response when asked if she wanted to go to the toilet, but would often wet herself soon afterwards. One of her children recalled that when they were little, their mother always referred to the toilet as 'the smallest room' (in French 'le petit coin' — literally 'the little corner'). Once Mitra changed her question to *'Do you want to go to the smallest room?'*, accidents became far less frequent.

Family carers often know and recognise these expressions from the person's past, but sometimes we need to think back to an earlier period to recall them, as happened in Mitra's example. More generally, we need to bear in mind that someone's age and background will influence how they speak, and also that they may well revert to earlier habits. As Bohling points out, when we are trying to fill in the fragments spoken by someone with Alzheimer's, we should keep in mind that the missing words may belong to a saying that was current when they were young.

> • *Ask yourself, is this unfamiliar word or expression one that was current in their past?*

KEEP LISTENING — WORDS ARE RARELY MEANINGLESS

It may not always be possible to make much sense of what someone with Alzheimer's is saying to you, but keep trying. Bear in mind that words are rarely completely meaningless, even if they are spoken by someone in an advanced stage of dementia. Don't be put off by the way some books on dementia treat what these people say as 'meaningless', 'nonsensical', 'confused' or a mere 'verbal salad'. Plenty of people who have lived for years alongside people with Alzheimer's strongly reject this view.

To conclude this chapter on an encouraging note, here is a demonstration of the point that we can make sense of even apparently 'nonsensical' words if we know how to listen to them. This demonstration comes from Hollis Bohling's work on listening to people with Alzheimer's disease. What makes it especially interesting for us, is that Bohling is directly refuting the view that what these people say is 'meaningless'.

First, here is what someone with Alzheimer's said in response to being shown a button and asked to 'tell about this'. Bohling is quoting this reply from another study, in which it appears as an example of the 'nonsensical utterances' produced by such people when they are tested.

> 'Right yes, on a button, very pretty. Well a man, I used to when I uh, but nobody would hardly (unintelligible word) that. This has got two things. Very much. This you mean hold that back. Well it is a the first day of a child's doesn't carry it very good. An uh, but as time goes on it becomes a very (unintelligible word).'[xx]

Admittedly, at first reading, this does seem fairly meaningless. However, Bohling produces a second version to show how a 'sensitive listener' could manage to work out what the person was trying to say.

> Right yes, on a (shirt). Very pretty. Well a man I used to <u>know</u> when I uh, but nobody would hardly <u>care about</u> that. This <u>button</u> has got, uh, two things. Very (important). This <u>button</u> you (need to) hold that back. Well, it is the first day of <u>school for</u> a child's. She/He doesn't (button) it very good. An uh, but as time goes on it becomes a very <u>routine thing</u>. [xxi]

Note that Bohling is working on the assumption that there are close links between what the person actually says and what they are trying to say. This is a key strategy for making better sense of what someone with Alzheimer's is saying.

I have left Bohling's brackets and underlinings as these show the general types of link that have produced this second version. Words in brackets replace a closely associated word in the original. For example, Bohling has replaced the first 'button' with 'shirt'. Underlined words have been added to complete fragments to which they seem to belong. The example of 'the first day of <u>school</u>' is one that I mentioned earlier. Working from such links, Bohling has been able to interpret what the person was trying to say, despite not having the advantage of knowing more about them or the context in which they were being tested.

CHAPTER 6
UNDERSTANDING THEIR STORIES

WHAT THIS CHAPTER COVERS

In this chapter I deal with the stories that people with Alzheimer's tell about themselves. These can be particularly difficult to cope with unless we look beyond the fact that they simply aren't true and start recognising the purposes that they serve for their tellers. Once we understand them as attempts by the other person to maintain their threatened sense of identity and worth, it becomes easier to listen sympathetically and to respond positively to them.

WHY THE STORIES ARE OFTEN DIFFICULT TO LISTEN TO

A common symptom of Alzheimer's disease, and one that often bothers carers, is that the people tell stories about themselves that simply aren't true. At first they may be simply trying to cover up holes in their memory by making up something plausible. Eventually, though, they will claim to have done things that are clearly impossible, like my mother telling us about diving for fabulous treasure in the nearby lake, climbing the mountain at night, being invited to the Royal Palace, and killing thousands of the enemy during the war. In the literature on dementia such story-telling is called **confabulation** or **pseudo-reminiscence**.

These more fantastic stories usually hang together as stories, but tend to be made up of a bewildering mixture of ingredients.

My mother's stories were typical in combining fact and fiction, past and present, far-off locations and ones nearby. One of her regular stories brought together her long-dead father, an event from her childhood in England (being made to climb up a church steeple), and the nearby mountain, which now became the setting for the new version of this event. As I mentioned earlier, one person or place in a story may be a combination of people and places. In this example the mountain, something tall and climbable in her immediate environment, had become the steeple from the past. Similarly, in another story, Willy the pet sheep, was made up of memories about the real Willy and about other pets that my mother had had or would like to have had.

Given their typical mixture of ingredients, it is no wonder that such stories should seem 'rambling' and 'confused'. Listening to them can be made even harder by the fact that they also tend to get endlessly repeated.

Once my mother got started on one of her favourite stories she could keep going for the rest of the morning, sometimes simply repeating the story but often making it more impressive — and fantastic — with each retelling. The letter of thanks that ended one story rapidly became a gold watch and ended up as ten gold watches and a whole heap of other treasures.

DON'T AUTOMATICALLY ASSUME A STORY IS UNTRUE

Some stories may be substantially true

Even though someone with Alzheimer's will be increasingly likely to tell fantastic stories, not all their stories will be untrue. Some of them may indeed fit the facts, and others, despite obvious inconsistencies, may well contain a solid core of truth.

In chapter 5 I quoted from my mother's account of her success at singing. This event happened much as she told me, although she improved slightly on some of the details to make the story better worth the telling. (This is perfectly normal — after all, we do tend to embroider the truth a bit when telling others about something that we have done!)

Another of my mother's regular stories was about being made especially welcome by shopkeepers and given some tangible token of their appreciation. Despite the fact that she sometimes told the story about shops she had never been into or that the tokens of appreciation were often improbably extravagant, the basic event was one that had indeed often happened in the past. Similarly, her claims about the work that she had done in the hospital garden were certainly true in relation to the many gardens that she had made earlier in her life.

Hence it is worth taking a moment to consider whether a story is actually true, or is closer to reality than may be immediately apparent. This prevents us underestimating the extent to which the person we care for may still be in touch with everyday reality. More importantly, it also ensures that we don't automatically dismiss their accounts of being neglected, exploited or abused in some way. Keep in mind the fact that someone with dementia is particularly vulnerable to being exploited, precisely because of their problems with memory and our tendency to dismiss whatever they do say as a delusion produced by their condition. Take the time to check whether the incident they've told you about did actually occur, even if on other occasions they may have simply imagined the event or have misinterpreted the absence of a long-gone object, say, as a recent theft.

However fantastic the story, the person isn't lying

We also need to realise that the more fantastic stories that they tell us are true too — at least for the teller. Even in her most amazing stories my mother was not intentionally lying to me — she really believed what she was saying. Because people with Alzheimer's lose the ability to distinguish between what they have done, what they have imagined, and what they may have come across on television or in a book, all their memories seem equally real to them.

RECOGNISE AND RESPOND TO THE PURPOSE BEHIND THE STORY

To listen sympathetically to stories that really do mix fact and fantasy, past and present, we have to stop worrying about the fact that they are literally untrue. Instead, we need to look beyond this and ask ourselves why the person is telling us this story — what general purposes does it serve? An important general strategy to help us answer this question is to look for the emotion behind the words, just as we do when listening to anything that someone with Alzheimer's is saying.

> - *Ask yourself, why are they telling me this? What purpose is this serving for them?*
>
> - *What feeling or idea does this story express?*

Storytelling as a means of interaction

Storytelling has the same overall purpose as conversation does — it is something that people do together, a means of social interaction.

> My mother had often in the past told me stories about her childhood. After she developed Alzheimer's disease, telling me stories about herself became one of her favourite activities. I would show that I was interested in what she was saying, and provide appropriate grunts, exclamations, comments and questions to encourage her to continue. We often spent a whole morning happily in this way.

Telling me a story about herself gave my mother two important roles — that of a storyteller with an appreciative listener and that of heroine in the stories that she told. Listening to her was valuable for me too, not only as a way of giving her pleasure, but also because her stories helped me to keep in touch with her subjective world.

'My story tells you that I am still someone of value'

The underlying purpose of many of my mother's stories was clearly to present herself as someone of value.

> She was boasting to me about something that she had achieved — climbing the unclimbable mountain, saving thousands of lives by having a notice put up warning people away from a dangerous thermal area, being invited to stay at the royal palace, slaying thousands of the enemy upon the nearby mountain top, being extravagantly rewarded for her custom by grateful shopkeepers.
>
> *'What do you think of that, Jane?'* my mother would demand at intervals, making it clear to me that I was supposed to be impressed. I would have achieved nothing by telling her that her story was literally untrue. Instead I responded as she was expecting me to, keeping in mind as I did so that she was enjoying telling me this story and that it had an important purpose to serve.

Through such stories my mother was presenting herself as active, powerful and appreciated. In so doing she was defending herself against the restrictions and powerlessness that old age and dementia had forced upon her. Indeed, her own comments often made this clear.

> On one occasion she told me with some triumph that she had slipped out of bed during the night, avoided being seen by the nurses on duty, and run up to the top of the mountain and back. The fact that she could now walk only with the help of elbow crutches made this exploit impossible, but was also the point of her story. As she remarked at the end of it, *'It's nice to know that there are some things that I can still do!'*

Presenting ourselves as someone of value is the underlying purpose of many of the stories that we tell about ourselves. From her study of the reminiscences of the normal elderly, Tarman concluded that many of these were basically designed to counteract the stigma associated with being old.[xxii] Being old and having Alzheimer's as well makes people even more vulnerable to being stigmatised, and thus even more in need of defending their threatened sense of self-worth.

> This is a point which my mother actually demonstrated during her story about receiving an invitation to the royal palace. She had been giving me details of the contents of the letter *'from the Queen'*, to prove the warmth of the invitation and to emphasise the pleasures that she — and I, as a close member of her family — would experience if we accepted it. She then added the following telling details about what happened when she received the letter.
>
> *'I thought to myself, "They'll see this letter, they'll think I'm doing something dreadful and probably, I don't know what I'm doing in — I'm really a villain and stealing things or …". So I took the letter to their head person and said, "I wish you'd — I'm sure your staff think that I'm not respectable and I'm not responsible for this letter. And this letter, it has just come through the post for me — I wish you would read it and return it to me at once." And then I went back a little later on and I said, "Well, did you read it?" And they said, "We're absolutely amazed and we know that you're not wrong at all and that it is a proper letter written from the royal palace at Windsor and it is addressed to you and it is a wonderful letter and we hope that you will go to Windsor when next you visit." '*

My mother could scarcely have made the point more explicitly. The letter from the palace has counteracted the bad opinion that she suspects the staff have of her, and they are now filled with proper amazement and respect.

- *Does the story suggest that the teller is still someone active and important?*

- *If so, show them that you appreciate their value as a person.*

Stories of wish-fulfilment

The royal palace story obviously also contains a strong element of wish-fulfilment. Instead of being stuck, semi-immobile amongst the residents in a nursing home, my mother has an invitation that will magic her away to a special place where she will be the centre of attention. Moreover, thanks to her influence, she can extend this rare treat to me and other members of her immediate family.

Many other carers have commented on the wish-fulfilment aspect of the fantasies of people with dementia. They recognise that the people they care for are reliving important and influential moments of their former lives, and often improving on the past.

My mother sometimes gave herself the extra children that she might have had if her subsequent pregnancies had been successful.

It may help you to accept such fantasies if you think of them as being shared dreams or daydreams. After all, most of us create imaginary pleasures and triumphs for ourselves at times in our daydreams, although we usually keep them to ourselves!

- *Does this story fulfil a secret wish?*

- *If so, think of your own daydreams and respond sympathetically.*

Claiming our sympathy

The stories that I have so far mentioned invite us to see the teller as someone important, deserving of our attention and respect. Other stories may make different claims, presenting the teller as someone who is threatened or unlucky or unhappy (for example) and therefore needing our sympathy.

> When my mother was first living in full-time residential care she told several visitors that she was terrified — someone or something terrible was creeping up on her or trying to get her.

The same basic strategy applies to these as to more boastful stories: identify the feeling being expressed and respond to that. The incident in the previous chapter of the woman at the day-care centre crying for her mother demonstrates how a particular carer did this.

> - *Ask yourself, is this story a way of asking for sympathy?*
>
> - *Respond sympathetically to the feelings being expressed*

Using one subject to talk about another — stories as metaphor

In the examples covered so far the meaning of the story or the emotion that it is expressing becomes reasonably obvious once we take the story at its face value instead of worrying about whether it is literally true or not. Some stories, however, may have more than one meaning. Although they have an obvious surface meaning, they seem to be telling us about something else as well. My mother's stories about someone or something terrible creeping up on her, for example, seem to be expressing her secret fears about what was happening to her. Another way of putting this is to say that the external threats that she was describing were acting as metaphors of the internal threat of her dementia.

Interestingly, we know that people with Alzheimer's have trouble with abstract ideas. However, the whole point about a metaphor is that it provides a concrete, tangible way of expressing something more general or abstract. Metaphors have been used to talk about one subject by means of another for thousands of years, as Aesop's fables and the parables in the Bible demonstrate. They are also extremely common in everyday speech. We say that someone's visit was 'a real breath of fresh air', for instance, or describe a smelly pair of socks as 'cheesy'. We also enjoy stories that have a double meaning, especially when the second meaning is a rude one. Indeed, metaphor is so much part of how we use language that it is hardly surprising to find it occurring in what people with Alzheimer's say.

Another of my mother's stories that has a second, metaphoric meaning is her account of the death of Willy, her pet sheep. This makes perfectly good sense as it stands. However, is it just about that? Or is telling me about Willy's death my mother's way of expressing her thoughts about what might lie in store for her? Many of the people with whom I have shared this story have, like me, seen it as a meditation on 'the good death' that we all secretly hope awaits us.

Here is my mother's description of Willy's death:

> 'Willy couldn't have had a more wonderful death than that very quick passing ... he'd got something the matter with him, and if he'd gone on he'd have been in considerable pain — but as it is he died peacefully and happily and if ever a sheep smiled it was Willy. And he did — he sort of died on my lap with a smile on his face, and I was stroking him.'
>
> When my mother was telling me this story on another occasion, she made clear that what she was saying about Willy could be applied to people too. 'He'd reached that stage where life was a burden. Like it would be for a person.'

Another example is my mother's story of walking in the distant hills looking for fragments of tapestry. To fill you in on the circumstances, my mother told us about this when she was already losing track of the details of her past life, but was still painfully aware of the fact. One thing that she did remember, and frequently spoke about at this time, was her mother's skill as a needlewoman.

> My mother stood by the window and pointed to the wooded hills on the horizon:
>
> 'All those different things — yet one doesn't notice how they fit together. I've walked up there looking for pieces of my mother's tapestry

> *— if you look closely you can see pieces of tapestry, some of them whole. I've gone for long walks across those hills looking for pieces, because they were worth a great deal to me.'*

> Literally this was nonsense — there were no pieces of my grandmother's tapestry up there, and my mother had never gone walking in those particular hills. However, given the background details that I have just shared with you, you will recognise, as we did, that the missing pieces of tapestry stand for the memories from the past that she had lost and was desperately trying to find again.

Tom Kitwood describes a very similar experience of someone with dementia finding a concrete way of speaking about their loss of memory:

> Peter talked, in a rather fragmented way, about his life. He could remember some parts of his distant past, but he had no memory at all for many of the more recent events. After some time Peter took me for a walk round the garden. He took me to some lattice-type fencing, and began to feel it with his fingers. He told me that the older fencing was very sound, but that some that had been put in recently was already rotting; he showed me an example, and crumbled a fragment in his fingers. I cannot prove it, but I felt sure that he was using this as a way of telling me about himself and his memory losses; it was like a repetition, in tangible terms, of our earlier conversation.[xxiii]

The possibility of the stories of people with dementia having this extra dimension of meaning is one that a number of other professional carers are finding extremely useful. Rik Cheston, for example, shows how we can increase our understanding of the stories told by people with dementia during reminiscence sessions if we take this dimension into account. Among the stories that he has collected is Roy's account of flying planes in Malaysia during the war. As Cheston points out, the details about the constant struggle to keep the airfields clear from the encroaching jungle have striking parallels with Roy's present struggle to keep his own memories safe. [xxiv]

- *Ask yourself, does this story have a second meaning?*

- *Does it express in some alternative, more concrete way thoughts or anxieties that are relevant to this person?*

THE VALUE OF RESPONDING SYMPATHETICALLY

Constructing an identity out of the fragments to hand

A more general way of understanding all these stories is to see them as attempts at constructing a valid history and identity out of whatever materials are still available. When someone with Alzheimer's tells us a personal story, they are engaging in something like the recycling of old clothes that happens when we do patchwork. Pieces from former garments are sewn together into something else — another skirt, a new waistcoat, perhaps, or a cushion cover — that suits our present needs. Thus, the person with Alzheimer's takes the surviving fragments of their memories of past people and events and combines these with details of their present life into a story about something that they have done.

Importantly, the events in the story usually happened 'here'.

> It was in the shop we were just passing that my mother had been recognised and rewarded; it was on the top of the mountain we could see *'just over there'* that she had slain so many enemies; it was this garden we were admiring that owed its beauty to her old skills as a gardener.

By locating these events within her present environment, my mother made her surroundings not only meaningful for her but also supportive of the history and identity that she was in the process of constructing.

The need for our sympathetic support

Someone with Alzheimer's is in danger of losing their social identity or self. This is not an inevitable effect of their disease; it is caused by other people refusing to recognise or value the identity to which they are laying claim. Hence it is extremely important that we understand the underlying purpose of the stories that people with Alzheimer's tell us about themselves. Instead of rejecting these stories because they don't fit the facts, we need to co-operate by responding to the unspoken plea that they are making: 'Listen to me, I am still a person, this is who I am, these are the things that I have done — and there are still things that I can do.'

CHAPTER 7

KEEPING IN TOUCH EVEN WHEN LIVING APART

WHAT THIS CHAPTER COVERS

In this chapter I consider some ways of managing to keep in touch when we are living apart from the person who has Alzheimer's disease. I have in mind two typical situations.

- *One is that the other person is living in some form of residential care. We may be living nearby, as my father was, but we are no longer spending all of our time together.*

- *The other situation is when we are absent for an extended period of time, whether this is due to our being away on a visit or to our living in a different town, or, as in my case, in a different country.*

Both of these circumstances are potential threats to our ability to keep in touch with the person for whom we care. However, there are various ways of counteracting these threats.

CHOOSING A HOME THAT WILL HELP YOU TO KEEP IN TOUCH

Some family carers manage to keep the person for whom they care at home right up to the end. However, there are many cases in which this is either not feasible or not in the best interests of the people concerned. Other obligations, or the health or other circumstances of would-be carers, the state of the person with dementia and their special requirements, and the past and present relationships within the family may make placement in residential care or a hospital inevitable. There are almost always feelings of guilt and anxiety about this, but carers have to accept that there are limits to what they can manage on their own. We have to work out what we can cope with, not just for a period of several days or a week but for an indeterminate number of years ahead. Staying well ourselves, so that we can continue to offer what help we can to the other person for as long as they need us, has to be our primary consideration.

One cause for concern if your family member is going to be placed in full-time professional care is how this will affect your relationship with them. When they are in care, will you still be able to keep in touch? The answer to this question will obviously depend to some extent on the care-giving establishment itself.

Closeness and accessibility are not the only criteria

A home's closeness to where you live, and possibly its accessibility by public transport, immediately present themselves as essential criteria. However, don't let yourself be entirely ruled by these considerations. The quality of care that a home offers and the quality of the ongoing involvement that it will let you have with your family member are even more important. Hence it is worth spending some time getting to know any place that you think might be suitable. You need to look beyond the mission statement in the entry, and the polite welcome and reassurances of staff towards a potential client, to what happens on a day-to-day basis. After all, both you and the person for whom you care may be spending a lot of time here in the future.

Basically what you will be trying to assess is whether this place is going to be a pleasant one to live in and to visit. This does not necessarily correlate with the size of the fees and the visible status of the establishment: I have encountered homes that I would have been happy to see my mother in at both ends of the scale.

The physical environment

If you are going to be living somewhere, you want it to feel homelike rather than institutional. Our nose is a good guide here — the smell of flowers and polish and something pleasant cooking are infinitely more welcoming than the rank odours of urine or cleaning fluid. Even though some residents are incontinent and an adequate level of hygiene has to be maintained, unpleasant smells like these are definitely a warning sign of inadequate care. They also discourage all but the most dedicated of visitors.

> I remember a woman whose husband was in care who rang me up in tears to ask if it was normal for a nursing home to smell of urine. This not only made her own visits unnecessarily stressful, but also made it impossible to take along the grandchildren — they had been so put off by the smell on their first visit that they refused to go again.

In larger residences it may be difficult to avoid all resemblance to a hospital or a hotel — especially in the corridors and service and reception areas. However, what about the bedrooms, dining room and lounges? Can bedrooms be made more personal by bringing in items of furniture and decorations from home? Do they look like bedrooms rather than hospital wards? Ideally the bedroom should provide a pleasant space where you can be together more privately at times when you prefer this.

Does the dining room look like somewhere you could enjoy eating, or does it seem tailored to the regimented feeding of people who can no longer feed themselves?

> I was happy to end a visit by escorting my mother to her place at her table. People were seated at tables of four, with some attempt made to put together reasonably compatible groups. The tables were neatly set and some effort was put in to how the food was presented and served. Despite the presence of a number of severely incapacitated people who needed to be spoon-fed, the overall atmosphere was that of a 'family-style' restaurant or tea-room. Meal times were positive events within each day.

Are the lounge areas for use rather than show? Are there cosy corners where your family member and his or her visitors can be comfortably intimate? It helps here if some of the chairs are light enough to be arranged to suit your group. The chairs obviously need to be easy to get in to and out of, but do they look like real home chairs or do they suggest rather too aggressively that anyone who will be sitting in them is likely to be incontinent? There are plenty of attractively patterned waterproof materials and water-resistant treatments available nowadays, so the old-fashioned, institutional plastic look is unnecessary.

If you are lucky, the overall style of the decor may be one that you and your family member can relate to. Some state-run hospital centres for people with dementia that I visited in the Bordeaux area of France made a point of using traditional regional furniture wherever possible, to give the facility a more familiar, homelike air.

The social environment

This is even more important than the physical environment, although if the surroundings have a pleasant feel to them this does indicate that the people running the place are trying to make it pleasant to live in. Look around you. Are things happening? Do most of the residents seem occupied or otherwise contented? Is there a program of activities in which people with dementia are encouraged to join and would you be welcome to join in too, if you wanted? Do staff take the time to stop and chat with residents, or are they always rushing about preoccupied with other priorities?

Bear in mind that a residential home, although it will often have some hospital facilities, is not a standard hospital. Instead of patients, it has long-term residents; their comfort and quality of life should therefore be the primary consideration.

A definite warning sign is seeing rather too many residents strapped into chairs and looking dopey — perhaps slumped in front of a television set. The current policy in professional care is that people with dementia should be treated as people, with kindness and respect. Physical and chemical restraints (strapping residents into chairs, and keeping them quiet by drugs) are now regarded as things to be used only as a last resort or in an emergency; they definitely should not be part of normal practice, or the standard way of dealing with so-called problem behaviours. In a home where residents are being treated as people — as individuals — the staff will make an effort to understand what is causing the problem behaviour and will try to find a more constructive solution.

> In a dementia care facility in a hospital that I visited in Belgium, one patient kept getting out of her chair and falling over. Instead of resorting to keeping her strapped in, staff wondered whether she was bored and simply trying to go somewhere more interesting. They installed her in a chair by the nursing station, where there was plenty of coming and going, and the problem disappeared.

If the home is a mixed one, including frail elderly and younger people with severe handicaps as well as people with dementia, are the people with dementia included in what is going on? Are they treated equally with other residents or do you get the impression that they are being less privileged, less valued? If they are confined to a separate area, how does it compare with the rest of the home?

How welcome you are made to feel is extremely important.

> I appreciated the fact that any visitors to the home where my mother was were automatically included in morning and afternoon tea. This came round on a trolley; tea was served in attractive cups and there was always some freshly prepared snack to go with it — an asparagus roll, perhaps, or a scone with jam and cream. Visitors were also welcome to share the main meals, although naturally the kitchen staff liked some notice of this and there was a modest charge.

Extremely important too is to feel that the nursing staff welcome you as a partner in care. They respect your personal knowledge of your family member, just as you respect their professional knowledge. I was extremely grateful for the readiness of the staff most closely involved with my mother to discuss aspects of her care and daily life with me. Having someone that you can talk to, who is sympathetic towards any concerns or anxieties that you may have, is invaluable for families of someone who is in care.

Providing for individual needs

I am thinking here not of medical needs so much as the special, human needs of the individuals living in a home.

> My mother had always enjoyed gardening. Being able to spend time out of doors, pottering about in a garden, continued to be one of her favourite ways of passing the time. We spent many happy hours together in the grounds of the residence where she was, and had our favourite private corner in it where we could sing loudly without disturbing other people.

Unfortunately, some homes would not have recognised this activity of my mother's as relevant, but labelled it as 'wandering'; in fact, some places actually tell you that they *don't take wanderers'*. A good home will have spaces indoors and out that are designed in such a way as to allow residents to walk about unaccompanied, and staff will recognise the benefits of this self-chosen exercise, rather than trying to prevent it.

You will know what are the special requirements of the person for whom you care and for your being able to keep in touch with them.

- If they are a practising member of a particular faith, access to the type of religious rituals that they are used to will be important for them.

- If they love animals, does the home have some resident pets?

- There may be an activity that has become central to maintaining your relationship — dancing together, or singing perhaps. Will it be easy for you to continue this?

- In some cases, being able to continue with the sexual side of your relationship may be relevant. Will staff be understanding and help you to have the appropriate privacy for this?

What happens when you drop in unexpectedly?

If you are thinking of buying a house, it is a good strategy to drop by unexpectedly to check whether the neighbourhood is really as pleasant as it seemed when you were taken to inspect the property. There may be rowdy neighbours or heavy traffic at certain times of day that nobody told you about. Dropping in unexpectedly is a good test of a potential residential home too. If they don't make you welcome whenever you visit as a potential customer, they are unlikely to make you welcome when you are already committed. Dropping in without warning gives you a chance to find out what the atmosphere is like at different times of day — are residents' different rhythms and preferences taken into account around washing and breakfast, for example, or is there a factory production-line approach? You can also drop in to coincide with some weekly activity that you feel will be valuable for your family member.

KEEPING IN TOUCH FROM A DISTANCE

From the time I left home I kept in touch with my parents through letters, postcards, phone calls and regular visits. As my mother's Alzheimer's developed, and especially after she had been admitted to full-time care, continuing to keep in touch with her became more of a challenge. I had to come up with some additional strategies to compensate for the effects of her memory problems and keep alive her impression of me as someone who still cared about her, even when I wasn't actually with her.

Tangible signs of our affection

One obvious strategy was to ensure that there were tangible signs of my affection for her to which my father and the staff of the home could draw her attention.

- Postcards were helpful here. If the latest one was tucked into the side of her mirror or propped up on her chest of drawers, visitors and staff would comment on it when they were in her room and read out the message to her. The fact that she had forgotten receiving the card was almost an advantage, because each fresh reading was like getting a new card from me.

- I also made a point of buying my mother some items of clothing that could serve as obvious reminders. The colourful wrap for wearing out of doors and the waistcoat that she often wore over her dress were known to have come from Australia and to be gifts from me. Comments such as *'I see you're wearing the wrap that Jane sent you from Australia'* reinforced the link between the garment and its absent giver.

I was dependent here upon the goodwill of my father and people in the home, but since they would be looking for something appropriate to say to my mother anyway, the cards and gifts of clothing were a ready-made topic for conversation.

- Photos and reminiscences about me were another means of reminding my mother of me in my absence. Indeed, my father found that retelling her the old family stories about some of the things I had got up to as a child was usually an excellent way of keeping her interested and entertained.

- Photographs were also a means of prolonging the effects of a visit from me. On one occasion my husband took a photograph of me and my mother sitting together in the front lounge, accompanied by Wally, her special friend, and we sent enlarged copies of this to both of them.

- Another strategy that I tried was sending my mother a 'talking' letter. Because reading more than a few words and making sense of them had become beyond her, I thought it was worth taping a personal message that she could listen to. In such messages I focused very much on things that we had done together and topics that we had talked about. As I did when we were together, I made sure in my talking letters that what I said presented her in a flattering light, stressing the importance that I placed on what she had said and done. Again, these talking letters depended for their success on someone being willing to play them for my mother, and reinforce my message through their own comments. However, this did provide my father with an activity that they could share.

Making the most of visits

Because I was living in another country, when I did visit it was usually for at least a week and often longer. As time got closer, the various people who knew that I was coming made a point of talking about this to my mother; indeed, a visit from me was another ready-made topic of conversation that they were glad to make use of.

> During my visits, I spent as much of each day with my mother as possible. I usually developed a routine that meshed into that of the home, so that I was sharing aspects of her daily life — the morning and afternoon teas, and the sing-along sessions, for example. We also had our own routine — walks and private singing sessions in the garden, playing with Growler and chatting together in the front lounge, washing Growler's head if he had had food dropped on it or inspecting my mother's clothes in her room if it was raining. The length of my visit and the routines that we developed increased the chances of my mother retaining some impression of my visit after I had left, especially when other people referred to it, as they obviously did.

Had my circumstances permitted I would have preferred being able to spend time with my mother on a much more regular basis. However, thanks partly to the strength and centrality of our relationship with each other and partly to the strategies that I have just outlined, I was able to keep in touch with her despite living at a distance.

CHAPTER 8
WHEN WORDS FAIL

WHAT THIS CHAPTER COVERS

In this chapter I suggest ways of coping when the other person either won't or can't speak to us any more, or their ability to speak is reduced to a bare minimum. Once again, we need to keep in mind the relevance of any interaction between us, no matter how minimal its content. Similarly, our presence and our voice may still be registering with them right at the end, even though they are no longer capable of responding to us.

SOME WORDS OF ENCOURAGEMENT

Helping to prolong the ability to speak

There are various ways in which you can help prolong the ability of someone with Alzheimer's to speak. Most importantly, the very fact that they are being spoken to and listened to with attention may well keep this ability alive. I am sure that this made a difference to my mother. Moreover, there are many instances of someone who has not uttered a word for weeks or even months starting to talk again in response to the right stimulus. Loic Laine and Marie Constaat, who ran memory workshops in Angers and in Paris, found that seeing and touching some familiar object from the past will provide the trigger to start normally silent people reminiscing.

People who are finding independent speech difficult can usually still come out with well-known songs and nursery rhymes.

My mother used the song 'Oh what a beautiful morning' to express her pleasure in an outing or a visit, and would sometimes adapt the words to suit the occasion. Until fairly late in her dementia she managed to astonish her listeners by her dramatic recitals of passages from Shakespeare and Tennyson that she had learnt by heart at school. When these were no longer accessible to her, she still enjoyed reciting nursery rhymes with us. Indeed, these became our major standby in the final months of her life.

The relevance of the emotion behind the words

We were fortunate in that my mother was able to speak reasonably clearly to us right up to the end, although her vocabulary was by then much reduced.

However, many other people in the final stages of Alzheimer's lose the ability to form intelligible words. Despite this, sympathetic listening should continue to help you to identify the general emotion behind what they are trying to say, especially given the additional clues provided by their body language and behaviour. Keep in mind that our emotions are an essential part of the meaning of what we say. Recognising that emotion, therefore, is a major step towards understanding the other person; it also tells us what sort of response we should be making to them.

Speaking and listening are always meaningful acts

Keep in mind too that the acts of speaking and listening are valuable in themselves. They have a basic meaning — I am making contact with you/I am responding to you — regardless of their actual content. Because of this, any act of speaking and listening is implicitly meaningful. This applies even if the other person is capable of no more than echoing the words said to them or repeating over and over the one apparently meaningless sound.

So do keep on speaking and listening to the person for whom you care. Even if you get no visible response, continue to speak to them nonetheless; for all you know, *your presence and your affection for them may be getting through to them even though they are unable to tell you so.*

WHEN WORDS FAIL

Thinking of sounds as a call sign

As I have already stressed, even if someone's ability to speak is reduced to the echoing of words or the repeating of a sound, this is still a meaningful act. It is helpful to think of such minimal sounds as a form of call sign. By echoing the word that we have just said to them, they are letting us know that they hear us. Similarly, the person who endlessly repeats *'dee dee dee dee dee'* is in effect signalling *'Here I am, respond to me'*, as some other signal, such as a hand stretched out towards us, often makes clear. They may have lost the power of speech, but they are reaching out to us and responding to us; they are trying to keep in touch as best they can.

Words are not the only means of responding

Don't forget either that words are not the only means of expressing oneself. As I said in chapter 3, we can communicate our feelings and interact with other people without a word being said. Gestures, facial expressions, how we stand or sit, and all the other resources of our body language contribute to any face-to-face interaction. Sometimes they replace words altogether. Being sensitive to these nonverbal signals is especially helpful in our interactions with someone who has Alzheimer's disease, and becomes increasingly so in the final stages. Many carers have known that their presence was still being felt, even at the very end, thanks to movements, grunts or a returned pressure of the hand.

Even silence and bad behaviour communicate something

Sometimes, though, the other person fails to respond, even though we are reasonably sure that they could if they really wanted to. Such a person may have their reasons for not responding, as Mitra Khosravi found out in the case of the woman who was being tested for dementia by the bearded professor (see chapter 2).

Someone with Alzheimer's disease rapidly loses whatever power or influence they may once have had in society or within their family. Refusing to respond to us may be one of the few ways in which they can still feel that they do have some degree of power.

Some instances of anti-social behaviour may have similar motives behind them. As Mitra says, violent words or gestures can be a form of self-assertion — a means of affirming that we exist, and that we

are still capable of doing something, even if it is something bad.[xxv]

She notes too that incontinence in someone who is normally continent can be a protest aimed at carers. One example that she gives is of a woman who expressed her annoyance at being shifted to another bedroom by urinating on the floor five times in an hour. Once Mitra took the time to explain to her why the change of room had been necessary, the problem stopped. Another example is a man who got rid of unwelcome visitors by the simple strategy of wetting himself.[xxvi]

BEING THERE AT THE END

As I have been stressing all along, the crucial thing is to continue with our efforts to get through to the other person. Simply by talking to them, by being actively there for them, we are showing them that someone still cares. Even though the person may be unable to respond to us, our being there may well be registering with them.

> Many years ago my husband spent three days in a coma, from which he was not expected to recover. However, I spent hours in the intensive care ward by his bedside talking to him; and I noticed that the nursing staff too spoke kindly to him and to all their other patients while they were attending to them. When my husband finally came to, he told us that for much of that time he had had the definite impression of being somewhere where he was being looked after.

At the very end, then, even if the person we care for is in a coma and expected to die soon, for all we know to the contrary we may still be getting through to them. Dr Marie-France Maugourd, a Paris-based psychologist specialising in helping terminal Alzheimer's patients and their families, speaks movingly of her experiences of family members around a deathbed continuing to talk to the person who is dying, each one summing up positive memories of that person and celebrating their past life. As she says, if anything of this gets through to the dying person it can only do them good, and the chance to express their feelings certainly benefits the other people present.

Some people suggest that the period of mourning for someone who had Alzheimer's disease begins well before their actual death, from the time their condition starts to make itself really felt. It is hard not to regret aspects of your past relationship which are no longer sustainable, but I cannot support this idea of premature mourning. The best that we can do for someone for whom we care is to continue to treat them as a person whom we love and value. This is incompatible with thinking of them as if they were already dead or partly dead. The years that may intervene between their diagnosis and their death are years of life to be lived, years when we can still be in touch.

My mother's death, when it came, was a relief. But the person whom I now mourn is the person whom I knew and loved for fifty-seven years, including those final years, with all the happy and sad memories of our times together.

A FINAL MESSAGE FROM GROWLER
— 'I LIKE BEING MADE A FUSS OF'

The last word belongs to Growler, my mother's teddy-bear companion and frequently her spokesperson. My mother is using her special growly voice to make clear that Growler is the one who is singing to her and me. The comments in brackets are my mother responding to Growler in her normal voice.

So I'm not so good as I could be

Oh how I wish that I was a little fatter

And I wish I was a little very much flatter.

Then I could go about and say how nicely I was out

And they'd think me much younger than I happen to be.

Oh I am older, and I don't get much attention

And the children run at me and laugh at me

And that's not really nice of them.

I like being made a fuss of

I love to be made a little fuss of

(And I make a fuss of you, don't I, Growler?)

On a cool and frosty morning.

(He loves a little bit of fuss.)

NOTES

[i] Kitwood T (1997): *Dementia Reconsidered.* Buckingham: Open University Press.

[ii] Sabat SR, Harre R (1992): The construction and deconstruction of self in Alzheimer's disease. *Ageing and Society* 12: 443–461

[iii] Gray-Davidson F (1995): *Alzheimer's, a Practical Guide.* London: Piatkus, pp. 80–81, 100.

[iv] Bayley J (1998): *Iris.* London: Duckworth.

[v] Garratt S, Hamilton-Smith E (1995): *Rethinking Dementia — an Australian Approach.* Melbourne: Ausmed Publications, p.124.

[vi] Naughtin G, Laidler T (1991): *When I Grow Too Old To Dream: Coping with Alzheimer's Disease.* North Blackburn: Collins Dove, p. 153.

[vii] Leech G (1981): *Semantics.* Harmondsworth: Penguin — see chapter 4 'Semantics and Society', pp. 40–58, for an accessible account of the functions of language, especially the phatic function.

[viii] Gray-Davidson F (1995): *Alzheimer's, a Practical Guide.* London: Piatkus, pp. 152–154.

[ix] Garratt S, Hamilton-Smith E (1995): *Rethinking Dementia — an Australian Approach.* Melbourne: Ausmed Publications, p.88.

[x] Khosravi M (1995): *La Vie Quotidienne du Malade d'Alzheimer.* Paris: Doin, p. 33 (my translation).

[xi] Smith B (1990): Role of Orientation Therapy and Reminiscence Therapy. In: Hamdy R (ed.) *Alzheimer's Disease: a Handbook for Caregivers.* St Louis: CV Mosby, p. 184.

[xii] Elery Hamilton-Smith and Sally Garratt, personal communication.

[xiii] Bohling HR (1991): Communication with Alzheimer's patients. *International Journal of Ageing and Human Development* 33 4: 249–267.

[xiv] Kitwood T (1997): *Dementia Reconsidered.* Buckingham: Open University Press, pp. 98–99.

xv Bohling (1991): Communication with Alzheimer's patients. *International Journal of Ageing and Human Development* 33 4: 256–257.

xvi Mitchell DB (1988): Memory and Language Deficits in Alzheimer's Disease. In: Dippel RL, Hutton JT (eds) *Caring for the Alzheimer Patient*. Buffalo/New York: Prometheus, pp. 81–97.

xvii Schwartz M, Marin OSM, Saffran EM (1979): Dissociation of language function in dementia; a case study. *Brain and Language* 7: 277–306.

xviii Elery Hamilton-Smith, personal communication.

xix Khosravi (1995): *La Vie Quotidienne du Malade d'Alzheimer*. Paris: Doin, p. 110.

xx Bohling (1991) Communication with Alzheimer's patients. *International Journal of Ageing and Human Development* 33 4: 252.

xxi Bohling (1991) Communication with Alzheimer's patients. *International Journal of Ageing and Human Development* 33 4: 253.

xxii Tarman VI (1988): Autobiography: the negotiation of a lifetime. *International Journal of Ageing and Human Development* 27: 171–191.

xxiii Kitwood T (1997): *Dementia Reconsidered*. Buckingham: Open University Press, p. 74.

xxiv Cheston R (1995): *PSIGE Newsletter* No. 24, pp. 35–36.

xxv Khosravi (1995): *La Vie Quotidienne du Malade d'Alzheimer*. Paris: Doin, p. 190.

xxvi Khosravi (1995): *La Vie Quotidienne du Malade d'Alzheimer*. Paris: Doin, p. 118.

INDEX